RUNAWAY TRAIN-
The Conductor Is Still On Board!

By
Sandra L. Kearse-Stockton, BSN, MHA and
Karmentrina S. Kearse, BS in Psychology, Minor in Diversity
Awareness

RUNAWAY TRAIN-
The Conductor Is Still On Board!

CONTENTS

INTRODUCTION

Welcome to a journey that aims to empower and inform those experiencing memory issues. In our golden years, it's not uncommon to face challenges with remembering names, appointments, or even day-to-day tasks. However, it's important to understand that struggling with memory does not signify the end of a fulfilling life.

Memory loss, while daunting, is a natural part of aging for many. For some, it might be mild forgetfulness, and for others, it could be more severe. Regardless of the degree, our intention with this book is to offer a comforting guide through the labyrinth of memory issues. We'll provide practical advice, valuable insights, and strategies to help manage and improve your memory. We aim to show you how to maintain your independence and quality of life.

In the pages that follow, you will find a wealth of information compiled with care and empathy. From understanding the inner workings of the aging brain to recognizing early signs of memory loss, this guide covers a comprehensive range of topics designed to address your concerns. Treatments, lifestyle adjustments, communication strategies, and more are discussed in detail, always with an emphasis on practicality and compassion.

Technology can be both a friend and a valuable tool in navigating memory issues. We'll explore various aids that can simplify your daily routines and enhance your cognitive skills. We'll also introduce you to support systems available to you, including family, friends, and professional groups.

Finally, we understand the emotional and psychological journey that accompanies memory concerns. This book is not just about addressing medical or practical aspects; it's about adopting a positive outlook on life. Embracing change and staying hopeful are crucial.

Let's embark on this enlightening path together, with trust and optimism, to show that memory issues are far from being a death sentence. They're merely a new chapter in the vibrant story of your life.

CHAPTER 1:
UNDERSTANDING MEMORY ISSUES

As we embrace the golden years of life, it's not uncommon to notice changes in our memory. While it can be unsettling, it's important to remember that experiencing memory issues doesn't mean we lose our sense of self or our ability to lead a fulfilling life. The aging brain undergoes natural alterations, and understanding these changes is the first step in managing and adapting to them. Memory challenges, though sometimes frustrating, are part of the broader tapestry of aging, and acknowledging them with patience and kindness can make a significant difference. By gaining insight into how our brains work as we age, and recognizing common memory problems, we empower ourselves to seek appropriate strategies and support, ensuring that these changes don't define us. This chapter will guide you through essential knowledge about memory issues, helping you to navigate this journey with confidence and resilience.

The Aging Brain

As we grow older, it's common to experience changes in various cognitive functions. One of the most profound changes occurs in our brain, impacting how we process, store, and retrieve information. The aging brain is a complex, intricate organ that undergoes a myriad of alterations over time. Understanding these changes can help us better manage the memory issues that come with age, providing us with a sense of control and reassurance.

The brain, much like any other part of the body, ages. Over the years, it faces natural wear and tear. The brain's ability to generate neurons decreases gradually. This doesn't necessarily translate to a severe decline in cognitive function straight away. Many individuals remain sharp and alert well into their later years. The variance in cognitive decline largely depends on several factors, including genetics, lifestyle, and overall health.

Neurotransmitters, the chemicals responsible for transmitting signals between neurons, also alter in an aging brain, affecting cognitive functions such as memory, focus, and processing speed. Changes in these neurotransmitters can play a role in why some older adults find it challenging to remember recent events or multitask effectively. The gradual depletion and less effective transmission of these chemicals can subtly impact memory over time.

It is also important to consider the brain's plasticity, or its ability to adapt and reorganize itself. Despite the aging process, the brain retains some degree of plasticity, enabling it to compensate for loss or damage. Engaging in mentally stimulating activities can promote neural connections and potentially slow cognitive decline. This, however, varies widely among individuals and is influenced by one's mental engagement throughout life.

Another aspect impacting the aging brain is the structural changes it undergoes. For instance, certain regions of the brain, such as the hippocampus, which is crucial for forming new memories, can shrink with age. While this can contribute to memory issues, it doesn't equate to an inevitable loss of all cognitive functions. Individuals can still live fulfilling lives, maintaining their independence and mental acuity by adopting various coping strategies.

Moreover, as we age, the brain's blood flow can decrease, further affecting cognitive functions. Less efficient circulation can mean fewer nutrients and oxygen reaching the brain, thereby influencing its ability to function at optimum levels. This highlights the importance of a healthy cardiovascular system for maintaining cognitive health in later years.

In addition, episodic memory, which involves recalling specific events or experiences, tends to be more affected by aging than semantic memory, the recall of general knowledge and facts. You might find it harder to remember the details of what you did last week but still recall the name of a state capital you learned about years ago. Variations in these types of memory can be frustrating but understanding these differences can help in developing strategies to manage them better.

While it's natural to experience some cognitive decline, significant memory issues are not an unavoidable part of aging. Many elderly individuals lead sharp and intellectually vibrant lives. Understanding and acknowledging the normal changes in the aging brain can help demystify the fear that often surrounds age-related cognitive decline. This awareness also reinforces that memory issues do not signify the end of one's ability to lead an active, engaging life.

Keeping the brain healthy and engaged through various activities can make a considerable difference. Activities such as reading, puzzles, volunteering, or even learning new skills can stimulate the brain and promote its health. Social interactions also play a critical role in maintaining cognitive health, providing mental stimulation and emotional support.

Healthy lifestyle choices, like a balanced diet, regular physical exercise, and sufficient sleep, contribute significantly to brain health. Physical activities improve blood circulation to the brain, and a nutrient-rich diet can provide the necessary fuel for optimal brain function. Adequate sleep is essential for memory consolidation and overall cognitive function. Skimping on sleep, especially in older age, can exacerbate memory issues and impair brain function.

Reducing stress is another crucial factor. Chronic stress can negatively impact the hippocampus, impairing memory and cognitive functions over time. Techniques such as mindfulness, meditation, or even simple breathing exercises can help manage stress, promoting better brain health.

Different coping mechanisms can also be useful in managing memory issues. Techniques like keeping a diary, using reminder notes, or setting alarms can help in daily functioning and mitigate the impact of memory lapses. Establishing routines and maintaining a consistent daily schedule can also provide a structure that supports memory function. These strategies not only help in managing memory issues but also enhance daily living quality.

Furthermore, maintaining an optimistic outlook can significantly enhance brain health. A positive attitude can inspire engagement in activities that stimulate the brain, promote social interactions, and encourage a proactive approach in managing health. An optimistic mindset can also reduce stress and increase overall resilience, thereby having a favorable impact on cognitive functions.

While the aging brain inevitably undergoes changes that can affect memory, it's essential to remember that these changes don't necessarily define one's capacity to live a full and enriching life. By understanding how the brain ages and taking proactive steps to support its health, memory issues can be managed effectively. With the right approach and mindset, it's entirely possible to navigate the complexities of the aging brain while maintaining a sense of independence and fulfillment.

In conclusion, the changes in the aging brain are natural and expected. By being mindful of these changes and adopting strategies to support cognitive health, you can continue to enjoy a robust mental life. Acknowledge the alterations, understand their impact, and embrace the tools and resources that aid in managing memory issues.

This approach can transform the way we perceive aging, viewing it not as a decline but as an opportunity to adapt and thrive.

Common Memory Problems

As we age, experiencing occasional memory lapses becomes part of life. You might forget where you placed your glasses or why you walked into a room. These are instances of common memory problems that many elders face. Such glitches are usually benign, but understanding them can alleviate much of the anxiety surrounding them.

The most frequent complaints include forgetting recent events, misplacing items, and difficulties recalling names or words. These minor lapses can be frustrating, but they're often part of normal aging. Let's delve a bit deeper into each of these issues to understand them better.

Forgetting recent events is probably the most noticeable concern. You might find it challenging to recall what you ate for breakfast or the name of a new acquaintance. This type of memory issue usually affects short-term memory and can be attributed to the brain's slower processing speed as we age.

Misplacing items like keys, glasses, or remote controls is another common problem. Often, the issue isn't that you've forgotten where you put the item, but rather that you didn't properly encode the location in your memory in the first place. Distractions and multitasking can contribute to this issue by affecting your ability to focus and remember.

Names and words can sometimes feel just out of reach. You might remember someone's face but not their name, or you could struggle to find the right word during a conversation. This phenomenon, known as "tip-of-the-tongue" syndrome, can be particularly vexing. These instances are typically harmless, although frequent occurrences can be bothersome.

Let's not forget the annoyance of forgetting appointments or plans. While we've all missed an appointment or two, increased frequency can signal a need to adopt better organizational strategies. Calendar reminders, notes, or even electronic gadgets can assist in keeping track of important dates.

Difficulty following conversations or stories is another issue that surfaces. You might find it challenging to keep up with rapid discussions or remember details from a story someone is telling you. This can be linked to both memory and processing speed. It's common to need a moment to process information fully before it gets stored in memory.

Remember, while these issues are common, they're not indicative of a debilitating condition. Nonetheless, it's crucial to distinguish them from more severe memory problems that require medical attention.

One common cause of concern is when individuals start to rely more heavily on memory aids. There's absolutely no shame in this; however, it's essential to assess if dependence on these aids is growing stronger than usual. Making lists, using journals, or setting reminders is wise and practical because they help keep track of daily tasks, supplementing the brain's natural capabilities.

Frequent repetition of the same questions is another common memory issue. You might forget you already asked a question and end up repeating it to others. While this is usually benign, it can sometimes cause frustration in social settings, for both you and the listener. Awareness and employing gentle reminders can help mitigate the annoyance of repetition.

Recognizing faces but struggling with names often comes hand-in-hand with aging. This memory glitch specifically troubles the hippocampus, the part of the brain responsible for naming things.

Associating names with stories or attributes can be an effective trick for reinforcing memory.

Disorientation in familiar places occurs occasionally, too. You might find yourself momentarily confused about where you are or how to get to a destination you've frequented. Although disconcerting, these instances are not uncommon. Familiarizing yourself with landmarks or always carrying a map or GPS device can provide reassurance.

Additionally, we encounter difficulty with multitasking as a common problem. Managing several tasks simultaneously becomes challenging and easier to forget some steps or actions mid-task. Prioritizing tasks and focusing on one thing at a time can help alleviate this issue.

The stigma of admitting memory lapses often prevents many from seeking support or talking about their experiences. It's crucial to foster an environment where talking about these common memory problems is normalized. Sharing experiences with others who can relate often helps in not only understanding but also managing them.

While it is comforting to know these issues are common, always consider consulting a healthcare provider if you're concerned about the frequency or severity of memory lapses. Early intervention and accurate assessment can offer peace of mind and assist in managing more serious concerns.

Emphasizing awareness and acceptance of these common memory problems is fundamental. They're part and parcel of the aging process and by understanding and addressing them, we pave the way for a more confident and less anxious experience. Remember, it's about living fully and positively, embracing each moment, and cherishing the wisdom that comes with age.

CHAPTER 2:
EARLY SIGNS OF MEMORY LOSS

As we continue to navigate the intricacies of aging, it's important to recognize the subtle hints that memory loss may be creeping into our daily lives. You might find yourself forgetting appointments or misplacing items more frequently; perhaps repeating questions or struggling with finding the right words in conversations. These early signs can be unsettling, fostering a sense of confusion or frustration. However, understanding these initial symptoms is the first step toward addressing them effectively. By observing these changes with a compassionate and analytical eye, you can seek timely advice from healthcare professionals, ensuring that memory issues are managed with care and empathy. Remember, experiencing memory lapses doesn't necessarily mean losing your independence or quality of life; it's simply a prompt to seek the right support and strategies to maintain your cognitive health.

Recognizing the Symptoms

Memory loss can manifest in various ways, and it's essential to recognize the early symptoms to address them promptly. The early signs of memory loss often creep in gradually, making them easy to overlook. However, noticing these signs early can pave the way for effective interventions and support. Let's delve into the symptoms one might encounter.

One of the initial indicators of memory issues is repeating the same question or story within a short span of time. You might find yourself telling a story to your friend and then an hour later recounting the same tale, unaware that they've already heard it. This isn't just forgetfulness; it's a sign that your brain is struggling to retain recent information.

Another common symptom is misplacing everyday objects. Occasionally losing your keys is normal, but consistently finding them in odd places—like the refrigerator or bathroom cabinet—could be a red flag. It's not just about misplacing items but the frequency and the odd locations where you find them.

Difficulty in performing familiar tasks is another symptom to watch out for. Simple activities, like making a cup of coffee or following a recipe you've known for years, can become challenging. You might find yourself forgetting steps or doing things out of order. This confusion, especially in routine activities, is a telltale sign.

Language problems, specifically finding the right words, can also indicate early memory loss. You might struggle to name objects or people, even if they are very familiar to you. This can lead to pauses during conversations as you search for words, or replacing the word entirely with something generalized, like calling a watch a "hand clock."

Deterioration in spatial awareness is another symptom. You might find it hard to navigate familiar environments. Driving to a well-known location or even walking around your neighborhood could become confusing. Additionally, you might see a decrease in your ability to judge distances or recognize colors and contrasting elements, affecting your overall navigation.

Changes in mood and personality can also be a sign of memory problems. You might notice increased irritability, anxiety, or even depression. These emotional changes can stem from the frustration and embarrassment of not remembering things or processing information as you once did.

Another indicator is diminished ability to follow and join a conversation. You might find it hard to stay engaged in discussions, often forgetting what was just said or having trouble with the flow of dialogue. This can lead to withdrawing from social activities and isolating oneself because keeping up with conversations becomes mentally taxing.

Decreased or poor judgment is another sign to be mindful of. For instance, you might find it challenging to make decisions or solve problems like you used to. Handling finances is a common area where this symptom shows up noticeably. Making financial decisions, paying bills, or even understanding the value of money can become confusing.

Loss of initiative can also signify early memory loss. Activities and hobbies that you once enjoyed may no longer seem appealing. You might find yourself sitting idle more often or lacking the desire to start new projects or engage in social activities.

Difficulty planning and organizing is another symptom. Setting up schedules, managing multiple tasks, or even following plans can become overwhelming. A simple task list might appear daunting, making it hard to focus and complete tasks in an orderly fashion.

It's important to note that occasional forgetfulness is normal for everyone. Stress, lack of sleep, and other factors can affect your memory temporarily. However, if these symptoms persist and begin affecting your daily life, it's crucial to consult with a healthcare provider.

Recognizing these symptoms in yourself or a loved one can be unsettling, but it's the first step toward addressing the issue. Early detection allows for better management and more effective treatment options. It also opens the door to a support system, whether it's family, friends, or professional caregivers.

Facing memory challenges can feel isolating, but remember that you're not alone. Many seniors experience similar issues, and there are resources and strategies available to help manage and mitigate the impact of memory loss. Embracing these tools and seeking support can lead to a better quality of life and well-being.

On a final note, we must approach this topic with empathy and understanding. Memory changes are part of aging, but they don't define one's worth or capabilities. Recognizing the symptoms early lays a foundation for a proactive approach, empowering you to handle memory loss with grace and dignity.

Assessing Memory Issues

Identifying memory issues early on is crucial for managing and potentially mitigating their impact on daily life. The initial step in this process involves a thorough assessment of one's cognitive functioning. This doesn't only mean noting what you tend to forget but also understanding the patterns and frequency of memory lapses. It's important to consider if these incidents are isolated or if they happen regularly. This detailed observation helps paint a clearer picture of your memory health.

An effective way to start assessing memory issues is by keeping a memory journal. Dedicate a notebook to jot down instances when you forget items, appointments, or names. Over time, this record can reveal trends and provide valuable information that can be discussed with healthcare professionals. Additionally, involving close family members or friends in this observation process can offer insights you might not notice on your own. They might see patterns or behaviors that you are not aware of, lending a different perspective to your assessments.

Another critical step in assessing memory issues is taking note of your ability to perform routine tasks. Are you finding it increasingly difficult to follow recipes you've known for years? Do you struggle with managing finances or handling other basic tasks that used to be second nature? These practical examples can be telling indicators of memory decline. In addition, consider if you are experiencing difficulties with orientation, such as getting lost in familiar places or forgetting the way to familiar locations.

Your emotional state and mindset can also provide clues to potential memory problems. Pay attention to your mood and how it may affect your cognitive abilities. Depression, anxiety, and stress often exacerbate memory issues. Therefore, addressing emotional well-being might play an essential role in alleviating some cognitive difficulties. Simple steps like engaging in regular physical activity, maintaining a healthy diet, and ensuring proper sleep can significantly influence both mood and memory.

In the process of assessing memory issues, undergoing a series of cognitive tests can offer a more structured evaluation. These tests, often administered by neuropsychologists or specialized healthcare providers, can objectively measure various aspects of memory, attention, problem-solving abilities, and more. While these assessments might sound daunting, they can provide valuable benchmarks and guide further diagnostic assessments or interventions if needed.

Seeking professional help for a comprehensive assessment is another important step. Medical professionals can conduct thorough evaluations that include physical examinations, detailed patient histories, and perhaps imaging tests like MRI or CT scans to rule out other underlying conditions. They may also evaluate blood tests to check for deficiencies or other treatable conditions that might be causing memory problems. Collaborating with a healthcare provider ensures that all factors contributing to memory issues are considered and addressed appropriately.

Many seniors fear that recognizing and assessing memory issues means conceding to a debilitating future, but early identification allows for timely interventions that can slow progression and enhance quality of life. Addressing memory concerns head-on opens the door to numerous supportive resources and strategies tailored to your personal needs. This proactive approach can alleviate anxiety surrounding forgetfulness and underserved negative connotations associated with it.

Additionally, participating in support groups can be highly beneficial. Sharing experiences with others facing similar challenges can provide emotional support, practical tips, and encouragement. Often, these groups provide an invaluable sense of community, making the journey less isolating. Educational seminars and workshops focusing on cognitive health keep you informed about the latest research and strategies to manage memory issues effectively.

Regularly engaging in mentally stimulating activities is also crucial in maintaining cognitive well-being. Puzzles, games, reading, and even new hobbies can keep your brain active and engaged. Social interactions play a significant part too. Engaging in conversations, participating in group activities, or volunteering can provide the mental stimulation critical in maintaining cognitive functions.

Finally, technology can play a supporting role when assessing memory issues. Various apps and gadgets are designed to help track memory lapses and offer exercises to improve cognitive function. These tools not only assist in the assessment process but also in the subsequent management and improving cognitive health. However, these should be seen as complementary aids rather than replacements for professional evaluations and interventions.

Ultimately, assessing memory issues involves a comprehensive and holistic approach. By combining self-assessment, professional help, emotional support, and cognitive stimulation, you can effectively monitor and manage memory concerns. Recognizing early signs and understanding that it's a collaborative process between you, your loved ones, and healthcare providers can lead to more effective management and a higher quality of life. Always remember, early detection and proactive intervention are the keys to navigating memory challenges successfully.

CHAPTER 3:
DIAGNOSIS AND TESTING

In the journey towards addressing memory issues, proper diagnosis and testing stand as crucial first steps. Medical evaluations help determine whether changes in memory are part of normal aging or signs of something more significant. During these evaluations, healthcare providers will review your medical history, medications, and may conduct physical exams to rule out other underlying conditions. Additionally, cognitive tests, which measure memory, problem-solving skills, and other aspects of cognitive function, provide valuable insight into how memory issues are affecting daily life. These tests are designed to be straightforward and often involve simple tasks like recalling words or drawing shapes. By understanding the importance and process of diagnosis and testing, you can take confident steps with your healthcare provider to manage and plan for future care, ensuring a focus on maintaining the highest quality of life possible.

Medical Evaluations

Medical evaluations represent a pivotal step in the process of diagnosing and managing memory issues. These evaluations are designed to uncover the underlying causes of memory loss and provide a clear path forward for treatment and support. Understanding this process is essential for anyone facing memory challenges, as it offers a structured approach to identify and address cognitive concerns.

When you or a loved one begins to experience memory problems, the first step is often to schedule a comprehensive medical evaluation.

During this initial consultation, a healthcare provider will take a detailed medical history. They will ask about the onset and progression of memory issues, other existing health conditions, medications being taken, and family history related to cognitive disorders. This thorough history can provide valuable insights into potential causes of memory loss.

Physical examinations are also a crucial component of medical evaluations. A healthcare provider will conduct a comprehensive physical exam to rule out any physical factors that might be affecting memory. Conditions such as thyroid problems, vitamin deficiencies, and infections can often contribute to cognitive decline. Identifying and treating these conditions early can sometimes improve or even reverse memory problems.

Laboratory tests are another essential part of the diagnostic process. Blood tests can check for various issues that might be impacting cognitive function, such as electrolyte imbalances, liver function, kidney function, and glucose levels. These tests help to rule out conditions that might be easily treated and allow the healthcare provider to focus on more complex causes of memory loss if present.

Brain imaging is often recommended as part of a comprehensive medical evaluation. Techniques such as MRI (magnetic resonance imaging) or CT (computed tomography) scans can provide detailed images of the brain's structure. These images can reveal abnormalities such as tumors, bleeding, structural changes, or strokes, which can all contribute to memory issues. Understanding the physical state of the brain helps in forming a more accurate diagnosis.

It's also common for healthcare providers to recommend neuropsychological testing. These tests are designed to evaluate different cognitive functions, including memory, attention, language, and problem-solving skills. Neuropsychological tests can help pinpoint specific areas of cognitive decline and provide a baseline against which future changes can be measured. The results of these tests can guide treatment plans and strategies to manage memory problems.

In some cases, genetic testing may be suggested, especially if there is a strong family history of memory disorders like Alzheimer's disease. Identifying genetic markers can provide additional context for the diagnosis and help in understanding the potential risk factors. However, it is important to approach genetic testing with careful consideration and consultation with a healthcare professional, as the results can have significant emotional and social implications.

While undergoing medical evaluations, communication between the patient, family members, and healthcare providers is vital. It's important to ask questions and understand the rationale behind different tests and assessments. Keeping a detailed record of symptoms, test results, and doctor's recommendations can be incredibly helpful. This collaborative approach ensures that everyone is on the same page and working together towards a common goal.

One of the more nuanced aspects of medical evaluations is the assessment of mental health. Conditions such as depression, anxiety, and stress can significantly impact memory. A thorough mental health evaluation can determine if these conditions are present, contributing to cognitive issues, or even mistaken for memory disorders. Treating mental health conditions can result in noticeable improvements in memory and overall cognitive function.

For those experiencing more subtle or early-stage memory issues, medical evaluations might also include lifestyle assessments. Evaluating factors such as diet, exercise, sleep patterns, and social interactions can provide a holistic view of what might be contributing to memory problems. Small lifestyle adjustments can sometimes yield significant improvements in cognitive health.

Another critical aspect of medical evaluations is the creation of a comprehensive care plan. This plan outlines the steps to be taken following the diagnosis, including treatments, lifestyle adjustments, and follow-up appointments. The care plan should be tailored to each individual's needs and regularly updated based on changes in symptoms and new information from ongoing evaluations.

Importantly, medical evaluations should be viewed as a continuous process rather than a one-time event. Regular follow-ups and reassessments allow healthcare providers to monitor progress, make necessary adjustments to treatment plans, and address any new or worsening symptoms promptly. This ongoing evaluation ensures that the approach to managing memory issues remains effective and personalized.

Facing memory issues can indeed be daunting, but understanding the role and process of medical evaluations can provide reassurance and a clear path forward. With thorough assessments and a collaborative approach, many underlying causes of memory problems can be identified and managed effectively. This proactive strategy not only improves quality of life but also empowers individuals and their families to navigate cognitive challenges with confidence and support.

Cognitive Tests

When addressing memory issues in older adults, cognitive tests play an essential role in the diagnostic process. These tests are designed to evaluate various mental functions, including memory, attention, language, and problem-solving skills. The aim is to identify cognitive impairments and determine their severity to tailor appropriate interventions. It's important to approach these tests with an open mind; they are tools to help understand one's cognitive health better.

Cognitive tests can be administered in multiple settings, such as a doctor's office, specialized clinics, or even at home for preliminary assessments. These tests vary from simple paper-and-pencil tasks to more advanced computerized assessments. Regardless of the method, the goal remains the same: to establish a clear picture of one's cognitive abilities. Many people find reassurance in knowing that these tests are non-invasive and usually free of discomfort.

One commonly used cognitive test is the Mini-Mental State Examination (MMSE). This brief, 30-point questionnaire measures various cognitive domains, including arithmetic, memory, and orientation. Though it's a quick screening tool, the MMSE provides valuable insights into cognitive functioning. For example, it might ask you to remember and later recall a short list of words, draw specific figures, or answer simple questions about the date and location.

Another frequently used test is the Montreal Cognitive Assessment (MoCA). It's slightly more comprehensive than the MMSE and covers additional areas such as executive function, language, and visuospatial abilities. The MoCA includes tasks like drawing a clock, naming animals, or following a set of instructions. These tasks might seem simple but are carefully designed to reveal underlying cognitive issues. The MoCA is particularly effective in detecting mild cognitive impairment, which other tests may miss.

Trail Making Tests (TMT) are also popular in cognitive evaluations. These tests consist of connecting a series of numbered and/or lettered circles in a specific order as quickly as possible. They help gauge visual attention and task-switching capabilities, offering another layer of understanding regarding cognitive ability. While they might just look like lines on paper, the patterns you create can tell a lot about how your brain is functioning.

Additional tests, such as the Clock Drawing Test and the Boston Naming Test, serve particular purposes. The Clock Drawing Test assesses visuospatial and executive functions by asking the individual to draw a clock showing a specific time. The Boston Naming Test evaluates language skills by having participants name pictures of common and uncommon objects. Each of these tests digs into different aspects of cognition, helping to construct a comprehensive cognitive profile.

Sometimes, healthcare providers might use computerized cognitive testing. These tests can offer real-time data and easier tracking of cognitive changes over time. They often include a broad array of tasks designed to test numerous cognitive functions. Having a digital record can make it easier to note subtle changes that might signal the onset of cognitive decline.

Neuropsychological testing is another cornerstone in cognitive assessment. Conducted by a trained neuropsychologist, these tests are extensive and may take several hours to complete. They delve into multiple cognitive areas with precision, offering a detailed and nuanced understanding of one's cognitive state. While these tests can be intense, their depth of detail helps in formulating a precise diagnosis and treatment plan.

Importantly, cognitive tests are not one-size-fits-all. The tests chosen often depend on the individual's specific symptoms and concerns. Some might need a broad overview of cognitive functionality, while others may require in-depth analysis in specific areas. The idea is to customize the testing to meet individual needs, ensuring the most accurate diagnosis.

After completing cognitive tests, it's crucial to review the results with a healthcare provider. Interpreting these results can be complex, involving multiple factors like educational background, cultural considerations, and even mood at the time of testing. A trained professional can help make sense of the scores and discuss the next steps, whether further testing is needed or it's time to consider treatment options.

It's natural to feel anxious about undergoing cognitive tests. After all, these tests touch on deeply personal abilities and can feel like a measure of one's worth. However, understanding that these assessments are merely tools to help guide better healthcare can alleviate some of this anxiety. They aim to improve your quality of life, not define you by your score.

For caregivers and family members, being supportive during this process is crucial. Encourage open discussions about feelings and fears related to cognitive testing. Your support can make a significant difference in how comfortable and willing an older adult feels about undergoing these evaluations. Remember, early detection through cognitive tests can lead to more effective management of memory issues.

In summary, cognitive tests are indispensable in diagnosing and managing memory issues. These evaluations provide a structured way to measure cognitive function, helping to pinpoint areas of concern and guiding the path toward effective treatment. Far from being a death sentence, understanding your cognitive health through these tests opens doors to interventions that can significantly improve your well-being and quality of life.

CHAPTER 4:
CAUSES OF MEMORY PROBLEMS

Memory problems can arise from a variety of causes, each influencing the way the brain stores and retrieves information. Medical conditions like Alzheimer's disease, other forms of dementia, and even strokes significantly impact memory function. However, we shouldn't overlook lifestyle factors such as chronic stress, poor diet, inadequate sleep, and lack of physical activity; these elements also play an essential role in cognitive health. Additionally, medications for other health issues might have side effects that affect memory. It's important to understand these diverse causes, as recognizing the source of memory problems can lead to appropriate and effective interventions. By addressing both medical conditions and lifestyle factors, seniors can take meaningful steps towards maintaining their cognitive abilities.

Medical Conditions

Memory problems don't just appear out of the blue; they often have underlying medical conditions that contribute to their onset. Understanding these conditions is the first step towards managing and improving memory issues. Early diagnosis and treatment of these medical conditions can sometimes make a significant difference, and knowledge of these causes can eliminate unnecessary worry.

One of the most common medical conditions causing memory problems is Alzheimer's Disease. Alzheimer's is a type of dementia that affects memory, thinking, and behavior. Symptoms eventually grow severe enough to interfere with daily tasks. Although age is the greatest known risk factor, Alzheimer's is not a normal part of aging. In its early stages, memory loss might seem like a minor forgetfulness, but it progressively worsens.

Another significant contributor to memory issues is vascular dementia, which occurs due to impaired blood flow to parts of the brain. This can be caused by a stroke or multiple small strokes over time. The damage left by these strokes can interrupt the flow of blood, preventing brain cells from getting the oxygen and nutrients they need. Symptoms vary, depending on the part of the brain affected, but can often include memory problems, confusion, and difficulty in concentrating.

Less commonly known but equally impactful are conditions such as Lewy body dementia and frontotemporal dementia. Lewy body dementia is characterized by abnormal protein deposits that disrupt brain functions. Symptoms can include fluctuations in attention and visual hallucinations, alongside memory loss. Frontotemporal dementia affects the frontal and temporal lobes of the brain, leading to changes in personality, behavior, and language, in addition to memory problems. Although these conditions are less common, their effects can be just as severe.

Beyond dementias, depression also plays a crucial role in memory issues, particularly in the elderly. Depression can cause memory problems and make it harder to concentrate. When someone is deeply troubled by emotional pain, the brain can become preoccupied, making it challenging to focus on daily tasks or recall simple information. Fortunately, addressing the root cause with medication or therapy can often improve memory.

An underactive thyroid, or hypothyroidism, is another condition that can lead to memory issues. The thyroid gland produces hormones that regulate metabolism. When it's sluggish, everything slows down, including brain function. Symptoms often include forgetfulness, fatigue, weight gain, and depression. The good news is that hypothyroidism can be treated with hormone replacement therapy, which often leads to significant improvements in memory function.

Infections and autoimmune diseases can also affect memory. Conditions such as multiple sclerosis, lupus, and HIV can cause systemic inflammation, which impacts brain function and memory. Treatment for these autoimmune diseases and infections often includes medications to manage the symptoms and reduce inflammation, potentially improving cognitive function.

Medications themselves can sometimes be the culprits. Certain drugs, especially those prescribed for insomnia, anxiety, or pain relief, can interfere with memory. Sedatives and tranquilizers, for example, may dampen brain activity to the point where remembering new information becomes difficult. It's vital to review all medications with a healthcare provider to see if adjustments or substitutions can be made to alleviate memory problems.

Chronic alcoholism is yet another condition that can contribute to memory issues. Alcohol affects the hippocampus, an area of the brain crucial for forming new memories. Over time, heavy drinking can lead to significant memory loss and even a condition known as Wernicke-Korsakoff syndrome, which is caused by a deficiency in vitamin B1. Fortunately, reducing alcohol intake and proper nutritional support can aid in recovery.

Neurological conditions such as epilepsy can also lead to memory challenges. Seizures can cause short- or long-term memory loss, depending on their frequency and severity. The parts of the brain involved in each seizure also play a role in the extent of memory impairment. Proper management of the condition with medication and lifestyle changes can greatly improve memory function in epileptic patients.

Sleep disorders, including sleep apnea and insomnia, have a direct impact on memory. When sleep is constantly interrupted, the brain doesn't have the opportunity to consolidate and save new information, making it difficult to recall past events. Treating sleep apnea with CPAP machines or addressing insomnia with behavioral therapies can often lead to significant improvements in memory.

Lastly, traumatic brain injuries (TBIs) from falls or accidents are another cause of memory problems. These injuries can damage brain cells and disrupt pathways important for memory. The severity of memory issues can vary based on the extent of the injury and the regions of the brain affected. Rehabilitation therapies, including physical and cognitive exercises, can help improve memory function following a TBI.

Understanding these medical conditions is crucial for managing memory problems effectively. While it's natural to feel worried about memory issues, it's important to remember that many of these underlying conditions can be treated or managed. With the right medical support and lifestyle adjustments, it's possible to improve memory function and maintain a high quality of life.

Lifestyle Factors

Our day-to-day habits have a significant influence on our cognitive health. Lifestyle factors, ranging from physical activity levels to social engagement, can either bolster or undermine our memory. In this section, we will explore how various lifestyle choices directly affect memory function, especially for the elderly. Understanding these factors can empower you to make informed decisions to enhance your memory and overall well-being.

Firstly, let's discuss physical activity. Regular exercise has been shown to have a positive impact on brain health. Physical activities, like walking, swimming, or yoga, increase blood flow to the brain, which can improve cognitive function. Not only does exercise boost mood and energy levels, but it also helps in maintaining a healthy weight. Being overweight or obese increases the risk of conditions like diabetes and hypertension, which are linked to memory problems.

A balanced diet is another cornerstone of cognitive health. Nutrition plays a critical role in brain function and memory. Diets rich in antioxidants, vitamins, and healthy fats help protect brain cells. Foods such as leafy greens, berries, nuts, whole grains, and fatty fish are particularly beneficial. Conversely, diets high in sugar and processed foods can lead to inflammation and damage to brain cells, subsequently impairing memory.

The role of social interaction cannot be understated. Engaging in regular social activities helps keep the brain active and engaged. Isolation and loneliness have been linked to cognitive decline and memory loss. Participating in community events, joining clubs, or simply keeping in touch with friends and family can provide the mental stimulation necessary to maintain memory function. Interestingly, activities that combine physical, mental, and social elements, such as dancing or group sports, offer a triple benefit.

Stress management is crucial for maintaining memory. Chronic stress releases hormones like cortisol, which can harm the brain over time. Practicing relaxation techniques such as meditation, deep breathing exercises, and mindfulness can reduce stress levels. Prioritizing leisure activities that bring joy and relaxation can also help. These strategies not only improve mental health but directly benefit cognitive function and memory.

Quality sleep is essential for memory consolidation. During deep sleep, the brain processes and stores information gathered throughout the day. Insufficient sleep can interfere with this process, leading to forgetfulness and difficulty concentrating. Establishing a regular sleep routine, creating a restful environment, and addressing sleep disorders are important steps in ensuring adequate rest.

Alcohol and tobacco use are lifestyle factors that can negatively impact memory. Excessive drinking can impair cognitive function and lead to long-term memory problems. Similarly, smoking has been linked to a higher risk of cognitive decline. Reducing or eliminating these substances can greatly improve brain health.

Another critical aspect is lifelong learning. Engaging in mental exercises and continuously challenging the brain can help maintain and improve memory. Activities such as reading, puzzles, learning a new skill or hobby, and even playing musical instruments stimulate the brain and keep it active. Enrolling in adult education courses or workshops can also provide the dual benefits of mental engagement and social interaction.

Routine and organization play vital roles in aiding memory. Establishing daily routines can help reduce the mental load, making it easier to remember tasks and responsibilities. Using calendars, planners, and various organizational tools can assist in keeping track of appointments and important dates. Creating specific places for essential items like keys and glasses ensures they are easily found when needed.

Regular health check-ups are necessary for early detection and management of conditions that might affect memory. Chronic conditions such as hypertension, diabetes, and high cholesterol significantly impact cognitive health if left unchecked. Working closely with healthcare providers to monitor and manage these conditions can mitigate the risk of memory issues.

In summary, multiple lifestyle factors can influence memory, especially as we age. By focusing on physical activity, nutrition, social interaction, stress management, sleep, and avoiding harmful substances, we can support our memory and improve our quality of life. Taking proactive steps in these areas empowers us to maintain cognitive health and leads to a more fulfilling, independent life. Addressing these aspects is not about implementing drastic changes but rather about making small, consistent adjustments that collectively make a significant difference.

Chapter 5:
Treatment Options

When it comes to handling memory issues, a plethora of treatment options exist that can make a significant difference in daily life. Medications prescribed by healthcare professionals can help manage symptoms and slow progression, while cognitive therapies aim to strengthen mental faculties through targeted exercises and activities. These treatments often work best when tailored to individual needs and combined with a holistic approach, including lifestyle adjustments. It is essential to consult with medical professionals to find the most effective strategy that addresses unique situations. Hope and improvement are not far off with the right combination of treatments, and each small step can lead to a better quality of life.

Medications

Managing memory issues often involves a multifaceted approach, one aspect of which can be the use of medications. It's important to know that while medications don't cure memory problems, they can help manage symptoms and improve quality of life. Knowing how these medications work and what to expect is crucial for both the individuals experiencing memory issues and their caregivers.

There are several types of medications commonly prescribed for memory-related conditions, particularly those targeting Alzheimer's disease and other forms of dementia. Acetylcholinesterase inhibitors, often simply called cholinesterase inhibitors, are one of the main classes of drugs used. These medications work by increasing levels of a neurotransmitter called acetylcholine, which is crucial for learning and memory. Drugs like donepezil, rivastigmine, and galantamine fall into this category and are often prescribed to slow the progression of symptoms.

Another category is the NMDA receptor antagonists, with memantine being the most notable. Memantine helps by regulating the activity of glutamate, another neurotransmitter involved in learning and memory. By balancing this neurotransmitter, memantine can help improve cognitive function and the ability to perform daily activities.

However, it's essential to understand that medications come with their own set of potential side effects. These can range from mild issues like nausea and dizziness to more severe reactions such as heart problems or even agitation. Regular monitoring by healthcare providers is critical to managing these side effects effectively. Communication between patients, family members, and healthcare providers can help in identifying any adverse reactions early.

Beyond traditional medications, there are also newer treatments under research. Some emerging therapies focus on beta-amyloid plaques, which are proteins that accumulate in the brains of those with Alzheimer's. Drugs targeting these plaques aim to reduce or prevent their formation, but they are still undergoing clinical trials. These experimental treatments offer hope for more effective management in the future but come with the caveat of being inaccessible at present until proven safe and effective.

For those experiencing co-occurring emotional or psychological symptoms like depression or anxiety, antidepressants or antipsychotic medications might also be used. Often, these medications aren't meant to improve memory directly but rather to manage symptoms that can exacerbate memory problems. Mood stabilizers and anti-anxiety medications can offer significant relief, allowing individuals to focus better and participate more fully in daily activities, which indirectly supports cognitive health.

When discussing medications, it's also vital to consider the role of over-the-counter (OTC) supplements. Many products marketed as "memory enhancers" are available without a prescription. However, the scientific evidence supporting their effectiveness is often limited. Supplements like ginkgo biloba, omega-3 fatty acids, and vitamin E are commonly discussed, yet they should be approached with caution and always under the guidance of a healthcare provider.

Furthermore, it's crucial to integrate medication management into a broader treatment plan that includes lifestyle adjustments and cognitive therapies. Medications can ease symptoms and provide a foundation for other types of interventions to be more effective.

The timing and dosage of medications can significantly impact their effectiveness. Some drugs may work better when taken at specific times of the day or perhaps with food. Adherence to prescribed schedules ensures the maximum benefit while minimizing potential side effects. Using pill organizers or setting reminders can be especially helpful in maintaining a consistent medication routine, contributing to better overall management of memory issues.

It's vital to continuously evaluate the effectiveness of medications. This process often involves regular appointments with healthcare providers to assess changes in symptoms and any side effects. Adjustments in dosages or even switching to different medications might be necessary based on individual responses. Open communication with caregivers and medical professionals is key to navigating these adjustments smoothly and ensuring that everyone is on the same page regarding the treatment plan.

Finally, it's worth mentioning that advances in pharmacogenomics—the study of how genes affect a person's response to drugs—offer a glimpse into the future of personalized medicine. Through genetic testing, we may soon be able to predict more accurately how different individuals will respond to various medications, thus paving the way for more customized and effective treatments for memory issues.

In summary, while medications for memory problems don't provide a cure, they play a crucial role in managing symptoms and improving the quality of life. Understanding how these medications work, their potential side effects, and the importance of adherence and regular monitoring can empower both patients and caregivers to make informed decisions about their treatment options. When combined with other therapies and lifestyle changes, medications can be a valuable part of a comprehensive approach to managing memory issues.

Cognitive Therapies

When it comes to addressing memory issues, cognitive therapies offer a beacon of hope. These therapies focus on enhancing cognitive function through a series of structured exercises and activities. By engaging the mind in targeted ways, seniors can experience significant improvements in their cognitive abilities, slowing the progression of memory issues. Moreover, cognitive therapies can be tailored to fit individual needs, making them highly adaptable and effective for a wide range of memory concerns.

One of the primary goals of cognitive therapy is to help individuals develop better mental strategies for processing information. For example, techniques such as "chunking" – breaking information into smaller, more manageable pieces – can be extremely beneficial. By learning to manage information more efficiently, seniors can often recall details with greater ease. The success of such strategies lies in their simplicity and the fact that they can be easily integrated into daily routines.

Memory recall exercises are another cornerstone of cognitive therapies. These exercises encourage the repeated practice of recalling information, which strengthens neural pathways associated with memory. Activities might include recalling a list of words, sequences of numbers, or specific details from stories. Over time, these exercises can help to reinforce memory patterns and make it easier to recall similar types of information in everyday life.

Engaging in activities that stimulate various parts of the brain is also crucial. Puzzles, word games, and even certain types of video games can activate different cognitive functions. These activities serve to keep the mind active and alert, enhancing not just memory, but also problem-solving skills and overall mental agility. Many seniors find these activities enjoyable, providing both cognitive and emotional benefits.

A key aspect of cognitive therapy is its adaptability. Therapists often work closely with their clients to tailor exercises and activities to their specific needs and abilities. For example, if a senior is struggling with remembering names, tailored exercises might focus on techniques for better name recall. This personalized approach increases the likelihood of success and helps to maintain motivation and engagement over time.

Cognitive therapies can also include more holistic practices such as mindfulness and meditation. These practices help individuals to focus their attention and enhance their awareness of the present moment. By reducing mental clutter and anxiety, mindfulness and meditation can indirectly improve memory function. They create a mental environment that is more conducive to clear thinking and recall.

Another beneficial component of cognitive therapy is cognitive-behavioral therapy (CBT). CBT helps individuals to challenge and change unhelpful thought patterns. For seniors dealing with memory issues, CBT can be particularly valuable. It can help reduce negative thoughts about memory loss, thereby reducing associated anxiety and depression. A more positive outlook can, in turn, facilitate better cognitive function.

The social aspect of cognitive therapies shouldn't be underestimated. Group therapy sessions, where participants engage in cognitive exercises together, can provide a sense of community and support. Social interaction itself is a powerful tool for cognitive stimulation. Engaging in discussions, sharing experiences, and supporting one another can create a dynamic environment that fosters cognitive improvement.

Technology also plays a vital role in modern cognitive therapies. There are numerous apps and digital tools designed to support cognitive health. These include brain training programs that offer a variety of exercises aimed at improving different cognitive functions. Such technology can be particularly appealing to those who are comfortable using digital devices, providing a flexible and accessible means of practicing cognitive exercises from the comfort of home.

It's important to note that consistency is key in cognitive therapies. Regular participation in cognitive exercises and activities promotes the best outcomes. Establishing a routine that incorporates these activities can help ensure that cognitive therapy becomes an enduring part of daily life. This consistency helps to reinforce the neural connections necessary for improved cognitive function.

While cognitive therapies are highly effective, they work best when integrated with other treatment options and lifestyle adjustments. Proper nutrition, regular physical exercise, and sufficient sleep all play essential roles in supporting cognitive health. By addressing memory issues holistically, seniors can maximize the benefits of cognitive therapy and promote overall well-being.

Additionally, family involvement can enhance the effectiveness of cognitive therapies. When family members participate in cognitive exercises or help to facilitate them, it strengthens the support system and reinforces positive behaviors. Family engagement can also provide additional emotional support, which is crucial for maintaining motivation and encouraging ongoing participation in cognitive practices.

In conclusion, cognitive therapies offer a powerful approach to managing memory issues. They provide practical tools and strategies that can improve cognitive function and quality of life for seniors. By integrating cognitive exercises into daily routines, maintaining a consistent practice, and involving loved ones in the process, seniors can take proactive steps toward preserving and enhancing their memory. Cognitive therapies remind us that, with the right support and dedication, maintaining mental sharpness and vitality is entirely within reach, even in our later years.

CHAPTER 6:
LIFESTYLE ADJUSTMENTS

As we navigate our journey with memory issues, it's crucial to consider the positive changes we can make in our daily lives. Lifestyle adjustments form a significant part of managing memory concerns effectively. A balanced diet, rich in nutrients that support brain health, alongside regular physical activity can make a world of difference. Prioritizing quality sleep and finding ways to manage stress can't be overstated—they help keep our minds sharp and spirits high. By tweaking various aspects of our routine, we empower ourselves to tackle memory challenges more robustly, embracing a proactive approach to our well-being.

Diet and Exercise

When it comes to addressing memory issues, diet and exercise play a pivotal role in one's lifestyle adjustments. These factors are particularly crucial for seniors experiencing memory decline, as they directly influence overall brain health. It's remarkable how small daily choices can create significant changes in cognitive function and general well-being.

Firstly, consider diet. What we consume has an undeniable impact on the brain. Studies have shown that diets rich in fruits, vegetables, lean proteins, and whole grains support cognitive function. Omega-3 fatty acids, found in fish like salmon and plant sources such as flaxseed, are known to promote brain health. Incorporating these into daily meals can be a game-changer for memory support.

On the contrary, it's wise to limit the intake of processed foods, sugars, and trans fats, which can exacerbate memory problems. Consuming too many of these can lead to inflammation and oxidative stress, both detrimental to cognitive health. Instead, pivot toward a Mediterranean-style diet, which emphasizes healthy fats, fresh produce, and seafood. It's not just beneficial for the heart; it's a boon for the brain as well.

Hydration is another often-overlooked aspect of a proper diet. Our brains are highly dependent on adequate water intake. Dehydration can lead to confusion, sluggish thinking, and memory lapses. Seniors should aim to drink plenty of water throughout the day, adjusting for any medications that might impact hydration levels.

Beyond what we eat, when we eat also matters. Regular meal times and portion control can help maintain steady blood sugar levels, which is crucial for brain function. Skipping meals or overeating can lead to spikes and drops in blood sugar, creating periods of fatigue and alertness that can confuse the body's natural rhythms and impact memory.

Now, let's talk about exercise. Physical activity is not just for maintaining a healthy weight or muscle strength; it's vital for brain health too. Regular exercise increases blood flow to the brain, promoting new neural connections and reducing the risk of developing memory-related issues. Activities such as walking, swimming, or even gentle stretching can be immensely beneficial.

It's important to find an exercise routine that's enjoyable and sustainable. Building a habit around physical activity often boils down to the enjoyment factor. Whether it's a morning walk in the park, a yoga class, or dancing to favorite tunes in the living room, the key is consistency. Even moderate exercise for 30 minutes a day can make a significant difference.

For those who may find traditional exercise challenging due to physical limitations, there are still plenty of options. Chair yoga, water aerobics, and light weightlifting can all provide the necessary movement without straining the body. The primary goal is to keep the body active, ensuring better blood flow and oxygen to the brain.

Strengthening activities are also crucial. Balance and coordination exercises, like tai chi, not only help maintain physical stability but also enhance mental sharpness. These exercises can prevent falls, which are a common concern for seniors, reducing the risk of injury and the resulting cognitive setbacks.

Combining physical exercise with mental exercise works wonders. Simple activities like gardening, which requires planning and physical effort, stimulate both body and mind. Group activities can also offer cognitive and social benefits, providing interaction that can reduce feelings of isolation and depression, further supporting memory function.

When integrating diet and exercise into daily routines, it's beneficial to set realistic and measurable goals. Small, incremental changes are often more sustainable and less overwhelming than drastic lifestyle overhauls. Keeping a journal to track meals and physical activity can provide a sense of accomplishment and help identify patterns or areas that need adjustment.

It's also helpful to engage loved ones in these lifestyle adjustments. Sharing meals rich in brain-healthy nutrients and enjoying joint exercise activities can create supportive environments that encourage adherence to these positive changes. Moreover, social interaction itself is a critical component of brain health; staying connected with friends and family can stave off memory decline.

While it may seem like a lot to consider, remember that every step toward a healthier diet and regular exercise routine is a step toward better memory care. It's about enhancing quality of life and maintaining the strength of both body and mind.

Creating these new habits may take time, but the rewards—greater clarity, enhanced memory function, and an improved sense of well-being—are well worth the effort. Diet and exercise are not just about adding years to life but about adding life to years, making every moment more precious and fulfilling.

Sleep and Stress Management

As we journey through life, the importance of restful sleep and effective stress management cannot be overstated, especially in our golden years. The two are deeply intertwined and play a critical role in cognitive function, emotional well-being, and overall health. By dedicating attention to these vital areas, we can make meaningful strides in preserving and enhancing our memory capabilities.

Sleep is the body's natural mechanism for restoration. During deep sleep stages, our brain engages in crucial processes such as consolidating memories, clearing out toxins, and repairing cells. Research has shown that disruptions in sleep patterns, whether from insomnia, sleep apnea, or restless leg syndrome, can have a profound impact on memory formation and recall. It's not just about the quantity but also the quality of sleep. Achieving restorative sleep involves creating a peaceful and conducive environment in the bedroom. This means a comfortable mattress, minimal noise, and a dark, cool room. It might be helpful to develop a pre-sleep routine that serves as a signal to your body that it is time to wind down.

Engaging in activities such as reading a book, listening to calming music, or practicing relaxation exercises can help prepare your mind and body for restful sleep. Avoiding stimulants like caffeine and heavy meals close to bedtime can also significantly improve sleep quality. Equally important, try to stick to a consistent sleep schedule, even on weekends. Your body thrives on routine, and a regular sleep pattern can enhance the regenerative aspects of sleep.

Stress, a common companion in modern life, can sneak up on us, especially during challenging times. While a certain level of stress is inevitable, chronic stress can wreak havoc on memory and cognitive function. When we are stressed, our body releases cortisol, a hormone that, in large quantities over sustained periods, can damage brain cells, particularly in the regions responsible for memory. Thus, effective stress management strategies are essential for maintaining cognitive health.

One powerful way to manage stress is through mindfulness and meditation practices. These practices have been shown to reduce stress hormones, increase gray matter in the brain, and even improve areas involved in memory and executive function. Starting with just a few minutes of meditation each day can build resilience against stress. Techniques such as deep breathing exercises, progressive muscle relaxation, and guided imagery can also be tremendously beneficial. There's no one-size-fits-all approach here; the key is finding what works best for you.

Physical activity is another excellent tool for managing stress. Regular exercise not only keeps the body healthy but also releases endorphins, the body's natural mood elevators. Whether it's a brisk walk in the park, gentle yoga, or tai chi, incorporating some form of physical activity into your daily routine can greatly reduce stress levels and, in turn, protect your memory health.

Social connections play a significant role as well. Engaging with family and friends provides emotional support and can act as a buffer against stress. Joining clubs, participating in group activities, or simply staying in touch with loved ones over a call or video chat can foster a sense of belonging and alleviate feelings of isolation, which can be a significant source of stress for the elderly.

Nutrition shouldn't be overlooked when discussing stress management. A balanced diet rich in fruits, vegetables, lean proteins, and whole grains can influence your mood and stress levels. Regular meals and staying hydrated contribute to a stable internal environment, making it easier to cope with stress.

It's also worth exploring hobbies and activities that you find joyful and relaxing. Gardening, painting, knitting, or even bird-watching can provide a therapeutic escape from daily stressors. These activities can offer a sense of accomplishment and engagement, both of which are important for mental well-being.

Lastly, if stress or sleep problems persist, seeking professional help is a step in the right direction. There are many professionals specialized in sleep disorders and stress management who can provide personalized recommendations and treatments.

By concentrating on sleep and stress management, we make an investment in our cognitive health. These lifestyle adjustments aren't just about adding years to our life but adding life to our years. Ensuring restful sleep and effectively managing stress can give us the clarity and emotional stability to face each day with confidence, improving not only our memory but our quality of life as well.

In the following chapters, we will continue to explore other aspects of lifestyle adjustments, including diet and exercise, providing a comprehensive approach to managing memory issues in a holistic and sustainable manner.

CHAPTER 7:
COMMUNICATION STRATEGIES

Effective communication is essential for individuals facing memory challenges, as it fosters understanding and provides emotional support for both the individual and their loved ones. It's important to approach conversations with patience and empathy, allowing time for the person to process and respond. Simplifying language, using visual aids, and gently repeating information can significantly aid comprehension. Establishing regular communication routines and engaging in active listening helps maintain clarity and reduces frustration. By nurturing positive interactions, one can create a supportive environment that enhances the quality of life for those navigating memory issues.

Talking with Family

Maintaining open lines of communication with your family can be one of the most effective strategies in managing memory issues. Facing memory problems can be daunting, and the feelings of frustration, anxiety, or even embarrassment are entirely natural. However, family members are often your strongest allies and understanding their role can foster a supportive environment.

Start by setting aside a quiet time to talk, free from distractions. It may be helpful to begin the conversation by sharing your experiences and feelings. Describe instances where memory lapses have affected your daily life. Be honest but gentle in your explanation. Clarity and openness can bridge the gap between what you're experiencing and how they can support you.

Your family members might have noticed changes over time too. Encourage them to share their observations. This exchange of viewpoints can provide a fuller picture of the situation, enabling everyone to work together more effectively. Remember, it's not about assigning blame but about understanding the collective impact of memory issues on the family unit.

Once you've shared your thoughts, it's crucial to listen to theirs. They might have a range of emotions, from concern to confusion, and giving them room to express these can foster a deeper mutual understanding. It's also an opportunity to dispel any myths or misconceptions they may have about memory problems.

Don't shy away from discussing practical aspects either. You might need their assistance with organizing medications, groceries, or even just reminding you of appointments. Creating a plan together, where everyone's role is outlined, can make daily life run more smoothly. For example, one family member might take charge of medical appointments while another handles the grocery shopping.

Adopting new communication strategies can also be beneficial. For instance, jotting down important points during conversations or using a shared calendar can help mitigate forgetfulness. Visual aids like sticky notes on the refrigerator or a bulletin board with daily tasks can be valuable tools.

Emotional support is equally important. Reassure your family that your memory issues don't define your entire being. The person they love is still very much present, deserving of respect and understanding. Sharing moments of joy, reminiscing about past experiences, and creating new memories can strengthen your bond, offering emotional sustenance for all involved.

Sometimes, family dynamics can make communication tricky. You may encounter resistance or disbelief, especially from those who aren't familiar with the nuances of memory issues. In such cases, involving a neutral third party, such as a counselor or a healthcare provider, might facilitate a more productive conversation. They can offer professional insights and guide the discussion in a constructive direction.

Equally significant is acknowledging and addressing the impact of your memory issues on your family members. They might have their own sets of fears and worries about your well-being. A conversation that includes their feelings and concerns can enhance mutual empathy and build a stronger support network.

It's also vital to keep these lines of communication open over time. Regular check-ins can ensure that everyone is coping well and can provide an opportunity to adjust the support plan as needed. Circumstances and needs may change, and staying adaptable is key to managing memory issues effectively.

Whether you realize it or not, your willingness to engage with your family about your memory issues sets a powerful precedent. It encourages an atmosphere of openness, where fears and uncertainties can be discussed freely. This atmosphere can help diminish the stigma often associated with memory problems, making it easier for future conversations.

Finally, remember to express gratitude. Acknowledging their support and efforts can go a long way in strengthening family bonds. Simple gestures like a thank-you note or a heartfelt conversation can convey your appreciation for their understanding and assistance.

Talking with family about memory issues can be challenging, but it is an essential step towards creating a supportive and understanding environment. With compassion, openness, and mutual respect, these discussions can lead to meaningful connections and a more manageable experience for everyone involved.

Speaking with Healthcare Providers

Engaging in meaningful conversations with healthcare providers can significantly impact the management of memory issues. It's beneficial to prepare for these interactions, ensuring you cover all necessary topics and concerns. A well-prepared discussion can lead to more accurate diagnoses, better treatment options, and an overall improved understanding of your condition.

Start by keeping a detailed record of your symptoms, including their frequency and severity. This information will provide valuable insight to your healthcare provider. Write down any specific instances where memory lapses have affected your daily life. Additionally, note any medications you're taking, including over-the-counter drugs and supplements, as some can impact cognitive functions.

When it's time for your appointment, consider bringing a trusted family member or friend. They can offer support, ask questions you might forget, and help remember the information provided by the healthcare provider. It's important to have someone who can advocate for you, especially if you're feeling overwhelmed or anxious during the consultation.

During the appointment, be honest and thorough in describing your memory issues. Don't minimize your experiences out of embarrassment or fear. Healthcare providers need a complete picture to offer the best possible care. Explain how these memory problems are affecting your everyday life, whether it's forgetting appointments, misplacing items, or difficulty following conversations.

Ask your healthcare provider specific questions to gain a deeper understanding of your condition and the steps that can be taken to manage it. Here are some questions you might consider:

- What could be causing my memory issues?

- Are there any lifestyle changes that may help improve my memory?

- What treatment options are available, and what are their potential side effects?

- What should I do if my symptoms worsen?

- How often should I have follow-up appointments?

It's also essential to discuss any emotional and psychological effects you're experiencing. Memory issues can lead to feelings of frustration, depression, or anxiety. These emotions are a normal response, but they should be openly communicated with your healthcare provider. They may recommend seeing a mental health professional or support group to help manage these feelings.

If you have any cognitive tests or screenings scheduled, ask your healthcare provider to explain the purpose of these tests and what they entail. Understanding the process can ease any anxiety you might have about the evaluations. Additionally, inquire about how to prepare for these tests to ensure accurate results.

Sometimes, the medical information provided can be overwhelming. Don't hesitate to request written materials or additional resources to review at home. Having these materials can help you digest the information at your own pace and come back with any follow-up questions during your next visit.

Building a good rapport with your healthcare provider is fundamental. Trust and open communication can make a significant difference in managing memory issues. If you feel your concerns are not being addressed, it's perfectly acceptable to seek a second opinion. Finding the right healthcare provider who listens and understands your needs is crucial for effective treatment and support.

Consider discussing advanced care planning with your healthcare provider. This can include topics like designating a healthcare proxy or making your wishes known regarding future healthcare decisions. While these conversations can be difficult, they are essential for ensuring that your preferences are respected in the event that your memory issues progress.

Remember, you are not alone in this journey. Healthcare providers are here to support you, and asking for help is a sign of strength. By preparing for your visits and maintaining open communication, you can navigate the challenges of memory issues with greater confidence and ease.

Following up after appointments is equally important. If new treatments or medications are prescribed, keep track of how they are affecting you and report any side effects. Regular updates with your healthcare provider can help fine-tune your treatment plan and ensure you're on the right path.

Lastly, don't forget to take care of yourself holistically. While medical interventions play a crucial role, integrating healthy lifestyle choices can also support cognitive health. Proper diet, exercise, and stress management are complementary to the treatments advised by your healthcare provider.

Open and honest communication with your healthcare providers is an invaluable tool in managing memory issues. It helps create a collaborative environment where both you and the healthcare team work towards the common goal of improving your quality of life. By taking an active role in your healthcare, you empower yourself to face the challenges of memory loss with resilience and optimism.

CHAPTER 8:
DAILY LIVING TIPS

Navigating the daily intricacies of life can be challenging, especially when dealing with memory issues. Creating structured routines and breaking tasks into manageable steps can significantly enhance your day-to-day living. Instead of feeling overwhelmed, focus on establishing a consistent schedule. Simple strategies like labeling household items, keeping essential objects in the same place, and using reminders can ease the strain on memory. It's also essential to stay physically active and socially engaged, as these activities help stimulate the brain. Remember, adapting to memory challenges is about finding what works best for you and embracing those methods to maintain a fulfilling and independent lifestyle.

Managing Tasks

Managing daily tasks can become increasingly challenging as memory issues arise, but it's far from impossible. With structured strategies and a touch of patience, you can maintain a sense of independence and accomplishment. Let's delve into practical methods to help you navigate daily responsibilities with greater ease.

Creating a Checklist: One of the most effective ways to manage tasks is by using checklists. Start your day by jotting down the tasks you need to accomplish. Prioritize them to ensure that the most important ones are dealt with first. This simple act of writing down your tasks can make them seem less daunting and provide a sense of direction.

Consider keeping your checklist in a prominent place, like on the refrigerator or a bulletin board. Using a pad of sticky notes or a dedicated notebook can also be beneficial. Digital options, such as apps on your smartphone or tablet, offer the advantage of reminders that can keep you on track throughout the day. The goal here is to make your to-do list a reliable anchor in your daily routine.

Breaking Tasks into Smaller Steps: Complex tasks can feel overwhelming, especially when memory issues are at play. Breaking them down into smaller, more manageable steps can make a significant difference. For example, rather than seeing "prepare lunch" as a single task, divide it into simpler steps such as "gather ingredients," "chop vegetables," and "cook pasta."

This method not only makes tasks feel more achievable but also provides a series of mini-accomplishments throughout the process. Each completed step builds momentum and fosters a greater sense of capability.

Using Visual Aids and Labels: Visual aids can be incredibly helpful in managing tasks. Labels on cabinets and drawers can guide you to the right places without having to rely solely on memory. Picture cues might also assist in recalling where items are stored or how appliances operate. You might use photos or images taped to cupboards to remind you where the coffee mugs or snacks are kept.

In addition to labels, consider using a calendar with large, easily readable dates. Mark important events, appointments, or tasks on this calendar to serve as daily visual reminders. These aids provide constant reinforcement, reducing the cognitive load on your memory.

Setting Up a Routine: Establishing a routine can bring a comforting structure to your daily life. A fixed schedule helps in reducing the cognitive effort required to remember various tasks, as activities become habitual over time. Consistent wake-up times, meal times, and bedtimes can anchor your day in predictability, making it easier to manage tasks around these constants.

When creating a routine, be realistic about your energy levels and capacities. Allow for flexibility where needed, but try to stick to the plan as much as possible. This regularity can provide both a psychological comfort and a practical framework for tackling daily activities.

Utilizing Alarms and Timers: Alarms and timers can serve as invaluable tools in managing both time and tasks. Use them to remind you when to start certain activities or when it's time to move on to the next task. For instance, set an alarm to remind you to take medications or start preparing dinner.

Timers can also keep you on track while performing tasks, ensuring that you don't spend too much or too little time on any one activity. Kitchen timers, clocks, or even apps designed to track intervals can be utilized effectively.

Delegating Tasks: It's important to recognize that you don't have to do everything yourself. Delegating tasks to family members or caregivers can lighten your load and reduce stress. Communicate openly about the areas where you need support, whether it's grocery shopping, house cleaning, or handling financial matters.

Involving others not only eases your burden but also fosters a sense of community and shared responsibility. Family and friends are usually more than willing to help; all it takes is asking.

Maintaining a Clean and Organized Environment: An orderly living space can significantly ease the process of managing tasks. Knowing exactly where items are located reduces the time and mental effort spent searching for them. Spend some time each week tidying up and organizing your home. This could include sorting mail, arranging kitchen ware, or putting away laundry promptly.

Clutter can be distracting and lead to misplaced items, so strive to keep your living area as neat as possible. This doesn't mean achieving perfection but maintaining a level of order that helps streamline your day-to-day activities.

Incorporating Technology Wisely: The modern world offers a plethora of technological aids designed to help manage tasks more efficiently. From smartphones and tablets to smart home devices, these tools can provide reminders, keep track of tasks, and even offer voice-activated assistance. Explore apps tailored for task management and memory aids. Many have user-friendly interfaces designed with simplicity in mind.

Voice-activated assistants like Alexa or Google Home can set reminders, play your favorite music, or find answers to your questions, all with simple voice commands. Incorporating these technologies can make managing daily tasks more intuitive and less labor-intensive.

Taking Breaks: Don't underestimate the value of breaks during your task management process. Taking a few moments to rest can rejuvenate your mind and body, making it easier to tackle the next task with renewed energy. A brief walk, some light stretching, or even a quiet moment with a cup of tea can do wonders.

Breaks prevent burnout and keep stress levels in check, allowing you to manage tasks more effectively over the course of the day.

Reflecting and Adapting: Lastly, take time to reflect on what strategies work best for you. Everyone is different, and what works for one person might not work for another. Assess your methods regularly and be open to adjustments. If something isn't working, don't hesitate to try a different strategy.

Managing tasks with memory issues requires patience, understanding, and a willingness to adapt. With the right tools and mindset, you can navigate daily tasks with confidence, preserving your independence and enhancing your quality of life. Remember, memory issues don't define your capabilities; they merely require a shift in approach. You are more than capable of achieving your daily goals, one task at a time.

Creating Routines

We all know that routines can be a stabilizing force in our lives. This is especially true for those among us facing memory issues. Establishing a daily routine can offer a sense of normalcy and control, helping to reduce anxiety and improve overall well-being. Creating a daily routine doesn't have to be complicated; even small, consistent habits can make a significant difference.

The first step in creating a routine is to identify the important activities that need to occur throughout your day. These include basic needs like eating, bathing, and sleeping. It is beneficial to keep these activities scheduled at the same time every day. For example, breakfast at 8 am, a morning walk at 9 am, and lunch at noon. Consistency helps reinforce memory through repetition and expectation.

While it might feel a bit restrictive at first, having a structured day can free your mind from the constant flux of decision-making. This can be particularly helpful for those who struggle with short-term memory issues. Benefits extend beyond mere convenience; having a set routine can help anchor your day and give a clear framework for what to expect. This stability can also make it easier for caregivers to assist and support where needed.

You don't need to fill every moment with activities. It's important to have windows of free time where you can relax, read, or engage in hobbies. Creating these pockets of free time within a structured day can provide a balanced approach, thereby improving your day-to-day experience. Think of your routine as a flexible guide rather than a strict schedule.

When setting up your routine, consider utilizing visual aids to remind you of the day's activities. A large calendar placed in a prominent location, such as the kitchen, can be an effective tool. Use bright colors or special markers to highlight key activities and appointments, making it easier to glance and remember. Notes and labels around the home can also serve as gentle reminders of daily tasks and appointments.

Technological aids can also be a great asset. Setting alarms on your phone or using a smart device like Alexa or Google Home can help remind you when it's time to take medication, eat meals, or perform other important activities. These tools can be customized to fit your specific routine and alert you with friendly reminders.

Another helpful approach is to create themed days to reduce the cognitive load of decision-making. For instance, designate specific days for certain activities: Monday could be for grocery shopping, Wednesday for laundry, and Friday for social activities or outings. This can simplify planning and add a layer of predictability to your week. Keep the theme days consistent, so they become second nature over time.

Don't overlook the importance of social interaction within your routine. Setting aside time to call or visit loved ones can greatly contribute to your emotional well-being and provide a much-needed break from solitary activities. Incorporate social engagements like family dinners, afternoon tea with friends, or even virtual calls into your weekly plan. These interactions offer support and help to keep feelings of loneliness at bay.

Exercise should also find its place within your daily routine. Whether it's a morning walk, stretching exercises, or a gentle yoga session, physical activity can be incredibly beneficial. Aim for simple, manageable exercise routines that can be done either at home or in your neighborhood. Regular exercise not only helps maintain physical health but also releases endorphins that can boost mood and cognitive function.

In the evening, it's time to wind down and prepare for a restful night. Establish a calming bedtime routine, like listening to soft music, reading a book, or practicing deep breathing exercises. Going to bed at the same time each night helps to create a strong sleep rhythm, which is crucial for better memory and cognitive function. A good night's sleep is foundational to your overall health and well-being.

When unexpected events occur, as they will, flexibility is key. It's okay to adapt your routine when necessary. If you miss an activity, don't be hard on yourself. Simply return to your routine as soon as possible. Consistency is beneficial, but so is being kind to yourself on the days when things don't go as planned.

To further enhance your routine, consider making it a family affair. Share your schedule with close family members or caregivers so they can provide support and encouragement. They can also help you stay on track and join you in daily activities, making routines more enjoyable. Being open about your routine with those around you creates a comprehensive support system that can make all the difference.

Creating a routine is not about rigidity but finding a rhythm that brings comfort and consistency to your daily life. Think of it as crafting a harmonious flow that nurtures both mind and body. Over time, these routines can become ingrained, offering a reliable framework that allows you to live each day with purpose and peace. Adjust as needed and always put your well-being at the forefront. This thoughtful approach to daily living can lead to a more fulfilled and peaceful existence, even in the face of memory challenges.

Remember, the goal isn't perfection but progress. Allow yourself the grace to grow into your new routines gradually. Embrace the process and recognize the positive changes that these small, yet significant, adjustments can bring to your life.

Chapter 9:
Technological Aids

As we navigate the challenges posed by memory issues, it's heartening to recognize the profound impact that technological aids can have on our daily lives. Advances in technology have introduced a range of tools specifically designed to assist with memory enhancement and management. From user-friendly apps that provide reminders for medication and appointments to innovative gadgets designed to locate misplaced items, these aids can seamlessly integrate into everyday routines. These tools don't just serve as simple convenience; they offer a tangible way to maintain independence and enhance the quality of life. With thoughtful use, any senior can leverage technology to stay organized, keep track of important tasks, and even stimulate cognitive functions through engaging activities. Innovatively designed for ease of use, these technological aids bring a sense of reassurance and empowerment, helping seniors to live more confidently and securely.

Memory-Enhancing Tools

In today's rapidly advancing world, technology has made significant strides in addressing various challenges, including memory issues. For seniors confronting memory loss, these technological tools can be both a lifeline and a source of independence. While confronting memory issues may seem daunting, a plethora of tools is available to support and enhance cognitive function, providing reassurance and practical assistance.

One of the most prevalent memory-enhancing tools is the digital calendar. Applications like Google Calendar or Apple Calendar allow seniors to set reminders for daily tasks, appointments, and medication schedules. These tools often sync across devices, ensuring reminders are accessible whether one is using a smartphone, tablet, or computer. The convenience of having timely prompts can alleviate the stress of remembering intricate schedules.

Voice-activated assistants, such as Amazon's Alexa and Google Assistant, also play a pivotal role in aiding memory. By simply issuing voice commands, users can set reminders, create shopping lists, and even find answers to pressing questions. These devices provide an intuitive and hands-free solution, particularly beneficial for those who may find traditional typing or writing cumbersome.

Moreover, digital notes are another invaluable tool. Applications like Evernote and Microsoft OneNote allow users to jot down important information quickly. These notes can be organized into categories, tagged for easy searchability, and synced across devices. This ensures that critical information is readily accessible whenever it's needed.

For those who are concerned about wandering or getting lost, GPS-enabled devices can provide peace of mind. Wearable technology, such as smartwatches or GPS trackers, can monitor a person's location and send alerts to caregivers if they venture beyond a predefined area. This technology not only helps ensure the safety of individuals but also provides a sense of freedom and confidence.

The realm of cognitive games and brain-training apps is another area where technology shines. Apps like Lumosity and BrainHQ offer a range of games designed to stimulate the brain and improve memory functions. These games adapt to the user's skill level, providing a customized experience that targets specific cognitive areas. Engaging in such activities daily can be as enjoyable as it is beneficial.

In addition, smart home systems can transform daily living by automating routine tasks. Devices such as smart thermostats, lights, and home security systems can be controlled via an app or voice command. By automating aspects of one's home environment, these tools reduce the cognitive load, allowing seniors to focus on more important or enjoyable activities.

Importantly, medication management systems have also evolved considerably. Pill dispensers that connect to mobile apps or devices can alert users when it's time to take their medication. These dispensers can be pre-filled and locked to ensure the correct dosage is taken. This addresses a common issue among seniors—forgetting to take medication or taking it incorrectly—which can have serious health implications.

Another promising development is the use of virtual reality (VR) for memory care. VR applications can immerse users in various experiences, from revisiting familiar places to exploring new environments. This can not only provide cognitive stimulation but also trigger memories and emotions that offer therapeutic benefits. While VR technology may still be emerging, its potential for enhancing memory care is vast.

Similarly, electronic personal assistants can help manage daily information. Services like RememberTheMilk or Todoist allow users to create detailed lists and tasks, ensuring nothing slips through the cracks. By integrating with other apps and devices, these services provide a seamless way to manage a multitude of daily demands.

Smartphone apps dedicated to health monitoring can also play an integral role. These apps can track everything from physical activity and sleep patterns to dietary intake and vital signs. By keeping detailed records, seniors can more easily share accurate health information with their healthcare providers, enabling better management of their conditions.

Moreover, innovative tools like the ReCoVRy game assist in memory rehabilitation. Developed specifically for those with memory concerns, such tools employ evidence-based techniques to enhance cognitive functions. Regular use can lead to noticeable improvements, providing users with a tangible sense of progress.

QR codes, though simple, are another tool that can support memory. By placing QR codes on daily items or important documents, users can scan them with a smartphone to retrieve detailed information, instructions, or reminders. This can be particularly useful for those who might forget the purpose of certain objects or the details of specific tasks.

Additionally, many of these memory-enhancing tools are customizable. Customization can range from adjusting the font size on a digital calendar to setting personalized alerts for medication dispensers. These adjustments ensure that the tools are as user-friendly and effective as possible for each individual's needs.

Importantly, while these technological aids provide robust support, their success largely depends on integration into daily routines and consistent use. It's essential for seniors, as well as their families and caregivers, to take the time to set up these tools properly and incorporate them into everyday life. Instructional guides or technical support services may also be beneficial to ensure seamless adoption.

In conclusion, memory-enhancing tools represent a powerful means to combat the challenges posed by memory issues. By leveraging the array of available technologies, seniors can maintain greater independence and quality of life. These tools not only aid memory but also offer emotional support and a sense of control, proving that memory issues are far from a death sentence. With the right technological aids, every day can be navigated with ease and confidence.

Apps and Gadgets

The rapid advancement of technology offers an array of apps and gadgets that can be a lifeline for those facing memory issues. These tools can greatly enhance the ability to manage day-to-day tasks, remember important events, and improve overall quality of life. In this section, we'll explore some of the most useful apps and gadgets tailored to help with memory retention and support.

To start, let's consider smartphone applications that are designed to assist with memory. These apps offer various functionalities, from setting reminders to providing cognitive exercises. For instance, there are apps like "Medisafe" which help you track your medication schedule. You can set alerts to remind you when it's time to take a pill, ensuring that you never miss a dose. Another notable mention is "Pillboxie," which offers a user-friendly interface where you can visualize your medications and receive timely notifications.

Equally impressive are apps that focus on cognitive training. "Lumosity" and "CogniFit" are two prominent examples, offering brain games that are specifically designed to improve memory, attention, and problem-solving skills. Regular use of these apps can contribute to maintaining and even enhancing cognitive abilities. These games are typically developed by neuroscientists and provide personalized training programs that adapt to your progress over time.

In addition to apps, wearable gadgets have become increasingly sophisticated. Take the Apple Watch, for instance. Beyond its fitness tracking capabilities, it can be an invaluable tool for those with memory concerns. Pairing it with reminder apps allows you to receive discreet vibrations on your wrist for important notifications, reducing the risk of forgetting essential tasks or appointments. Apple's "Health" app also promotes overall well-being by tracking various health metrics like heart rate and physical activity, offering a holistic view of one's health.

Voice-activated assistants like Amazon Alexa, Google Assistant, and Apple's Siri have transformative impacts as well. These devices can be stationed around your home and can be activated with a simple voice command. Whether you need to set a reminder, create a shopping list, or even call a loved one, these assistants are incredibly helpful. They offer a hands-free experience, which is particularly useful if you're prone to misplacing your phone or need assistance quickly.

Now, let's talk about GPS-based locating devices. If tendencies to lose personal items like keys or wallets are prevalent, gadgets like "Tile" or "TrackR" come to the rescue. These small devices can be attached to your belongings, and through a smartphone app, you can easily locate any lost item. Such innovations not only save time but also reduce the stress associated with losing important personal items.

A remarkable gadget in this space is the "Smartpen." Livescribe's various models of smartpens not only capture handwritten notes but also record audio that syncs with your written words. This can be particularly useful during medical appointments or important meetings. You can later play back what was said by tapping on your handwritten notes. It's like an all-in-one note-taking assistant, preventing any significant points from being missed.

Then there are smart home systems. These intelligent systems, such as those offered by Nest and other home automation providers, allow you to control various home elements from heating to security remotely. They can be scheduled to perform certain tasks at specific times or even send alerts to your phone, helping you keep track of household responsibilities and enhancing overall safety.

Let's not overlook the digital photo frames and smart displays that can help jog memory. Gadgets like "Nixplay" or digital frames supported by Google Photos allow loved ones to upload photos remotely. These rotating pictures can serve as gentle reminders of happy times and cherished moments, uplifting your spirits and reinforcing family bonds. In moments of feeling forgetful or lonely, seeing familiar faces and places can bring comfort and joy.

For those who enjoy reading but find it difficult to keep track of where they left off, e-readers like Amazon Kindle or apps like Audible for audiobooks provide solutions. Kindle devices allow for bookmarks, notes, and highlights, which can all be neatly organized and accessed later. Audiobooks, on the other hand, offer the experience of reading through listening, which can be particularly beneficial for those who find traditional reading challenging.

The advancements in AI have also led to the development of personal health monitors. Gadgets like "Fitbit" or "Garmin" watches not only count steps but can monitor your sleep patterns, detect abnormalities in heart rate, and offer insights into overall physical health. In syncing with their respective apps, they help create a comprehensive health profile that healthcare providers can find useful.

Finally, online platforms that facilitate connection and community should not be forgotten. Apps like "Nextdoor" connect you with your neighborhood, keeping you informed about local events or concerns. Social media platforms like Facebook have groups and pages dedicated to seniors dealing with memory issues. Such interactions can foster a sense of community and belonging, providing both emotional and social support through shared experiences.

In sum, apps and gadgets are more than just electronic tools; they serve as essential companions in managing memory issues. They provide the crucial support needed for carrying out daily responsibilities, offer cognitive stimulation to keep the mind sharp, and bridge the gap between physical and digital ways of living. Embracing these technological aids can transform many aspects of daily life, offering not only convenience but also peace of mind.

CHAPTER 10:
SUPPORT SYSTEMS

When faced with memory issues, knowing that you have reliable support systems can make a significant difference in your daily life. Family and friends play a crucial role by offering emotional support, helping with day-to-day tasks, and providing a stable environment that mitigates stress. Additionally, joining support groups can create a sense of community, allowing you to share experiences, learn from others, and discover effective coping strategies. These support networks are integral, offering not only practical assistance but also emotional and mental reinforcement that can greatly enhance your quality of life.

Family and Friends

As you navigate the choppy waters of memory issues, your family and friends are the sturdy ships that sail alongside you. They provide not only emotional support but also practical assistance, helping you maintain a higher quality of life. While memory problems can be isolating, the strong bonds you share with your loved ones can offer a safety net that catches you when you stumble.

At times, you may feel as though remembering names, faces, or even past experiences becomes an insurmountable challenge. Yet, amidst these struggles, familiar voices and gentle reassurances can ground you. Imagine having a conversation with a relative who reminds you of cherished memories or a friend who helps you recall a shared adventure. These interactions can be both comforting and invigorating, reminding you that you are never alone in your journey.

The intricate dance of daily life can become overwhelming when memory issues arise. Family members often step up to the plate, assuming roles you might find difficult to manage. They might assist in organizing your medications, setting reminders for appointments, or even helping with household chores. These acts of love and service, though sometimes small, contribute significantly to your overall well-being.

It's equally important to accept that your friends will play a different, yet complementary, role. They may take you out for a walk, engage in stimulating conversations, or simply offer companionship. Friends provide a sense of normalcy and a link to social activities, which become even more important as you navigate the complexities of memory loss.

Let's not overlook the emotional landscape. Family and friends provide a reservoir of emotional stability, which is crucial for mental health. They listen, offer advice, and provide a shoulder to lean on when things get tough. Engaging in open, heartfelt conversations about your memory struggles can foster understanding and empathy, deepening your connections.

Consider regular family gatherings or habitual coffee meet-ups with friends. These rituals can serve as anchors in your routine, giving you something to look forward to. Visual and sensory reminders from these gatherings—like the aroma of brewing coffee or the laughter of a grandchild—can create touchstones that help jog your memory.

It's also beneficial to involve your family in your treatment plan. Having them present during medical appointments ensures that they are well-informed about your condition and the recommended therapies. They're likely to remember details you might forget, making them valuable allies in your care management.

But what about misunderstandings or frustrations? Family and friends can sometimes struggle to understand the full scope of your experience. Patience is key here. As much as they're your support system, educating them about your condition can go a long way. This mutual understanding fosters a more nurturing and supportive environment for everyone involved.

Moreover, it's healthy to set boundaries. Having honest discussions about what you need—and what you don't need—can clarify expectations. For instance, if too much help feels suffocating, let them know you appreciate their support but also need some space to manage tasks independently.

Interdependence is the essence of this chapter on family and friends. While they offer you support, remember that your existence, your experiences, and wisdom, offer them immense value too. Your stories, advice, and love enrich their lives, creating a reciprocal relationship that benefits everyone.

If you ever feel like a burden, just take a moment to think about the close relationships you cherish. Visualize the smiles, the shared jokes, the warmth of a hug. Know that these connections are far more substantial than any illness. Love and friendship transcend boundaries, even the ones set by failing memory.

Family and friends also serve as advocates in scenarios where you might feel overwhelmed. Whether it's clarifying a doctor's instructions or dealing with legal paperwork, having someone by your side provides reassurance and counters the uncertainties that come with memory issues.

Financially, your family can assist in managing budgets, paying bills, and handling any other monetary responsibilities you may have.

A well-organized financial plan, often established with them, reduces stress and allows you to focus on your health and happiness.

Incorporate your loved ones into activities that stimulate the mind. Activities like puzzles, reading, or discussing current events can be shared experiences that offer both cognitive benefits and the joy of companionship. These joint activities can serve as a pleasant distraction from the daily struggles of memory loss.

Lastly, never underestimate the power of presence. Sometimes, family and friends don't have to say anything or do anything specific. Just being there, sharing the same space, can be incredibly comforting. A hug, a hand-held, or even sitting in silence together can speak volumes.

In summary, your family and friends are invaluable pillars of your support system. They contribute to your emotional, physical, and mental well-being, enriching your life in countless ways. Remember to lean on them, cherish them, and also to celebrate the love and warmth they bring into your life. With them by your side, facing memory issues becomes not just manageable, but a journey filled with hope, love, and shared strength.

Support Groups

Being part of a support group can make a substantial difference for seniors facing memory issues, offering both emotional solace and practical advice. In many cases, support group meetings can provide a welcoming environment where you can share your feelings and experiences without judgment. These gatherings can be a sanctuary, a place to feel understood and less isolated in the journey of coping with memory loss.

Support groups typically consist of individuals who are dealing with similar challenges, thus fostering an environment of empathy and shared understanding. You may meet people who are at different stages of memory decline, which can provide a spectrum of perspectives and coping strategies. The conversations in such settings often range from discussing medication side effects to simple tips for improving daily routines. The value of listening to others who have walked in your shoes cannot be overstated, as it can help validate your own experiences and offer a sense of normalcy in what might otherwise feel like a solitary struggle.

These groups often have a facilitator or leader who guides the discussion and ensures that everyone has an opportunity to speak. Facilitators are usually well-versed in the nuances of memory issues and offer both professional insights and emotional support. The structure of the meetings varies; some may follow a specific agenda while others allow for free-flowing conversation. Regardless, these gatherings function as a lifeline, offering you proof that you are not alone and that help is always within reach.

Another benefit of support groups is the wealth of practical advice that flows freely among members. For instance, someone may have discovered a useful app that helps with daily reminders, or another might share a technique for managing anxiety. These nuggets of wisdom, often born of personal experience, can be more impactful than generic advice found in books or online. Members tend to be very supportive and willing to share what has worked for them, making the journey easier to navigate.

The emotional support gained from these groups is invaluable. It can be incredibly comforting to express your fears, frustrations, and triumphs in a safe space. Just knowing that you're part of a community that truly understands what you're going through can alleviate some of the emotional burden. Many members find long-lasting friendships within these circles, adding another layer of support and camaraderie to their lives.

Moreover, support groups can provide family members and caregivers with essential insights. Some groups are open to loved ones, allowing them to learn, share, and understand the complexities of memory issues from a more informed perspective. These sessions can offer caregivers coping strategies, stress relief techniques, and even advice on how to better communicate with their loved ones. This shared understanding can strengthen familial bonds and improve the quality of care provided.

Resources for finding support groups are plentiful. Local communities often have senior centers or healthcare facilities that host regular meetings. These centers may offer both in-person and virtual options, catering to those who may find it difficult to travel or prefer the convenience of joining from home. Online databases and registries can also connect you with groups that meet your specific needs and schedules.

Some organizations specialize in support for various types of memory-related conditions. For example, groups focused on Alzheimer's disease are prevalent and offer targeted advice and support tailored to the unique challenges posed by this condition. Similarly, there are groups dedicated to other forms of dementia, each providing specialized knowledge and a sense of belonging.

Engaging with a support group can also motivate you to take proactive steps in managing your condition. As you hear stories of others facing similar challenges, you're likely to be inspired by their resilience and creativity. This newfound motivation can propel you to adopt new strategies and embrace positive changes in your own life. Sometimes, just seeing others persevere is enough to strengthen your resolve and encourage you to keep moving forward.

The consistency of meeting regularly with a group can also help you establish a routine. Regular gatherings offer a sense of stability and something to look forward to, which can be incredibly reassuring. This sense of routine can spill over into other areas of your life, assisting in the creation of more structured and manageable daily activities.

If you're hesitant about joining a support group, it's worth giving it a try at least once. Most groups are welcoming to newcomers and understand that it can be daunting to take that first step. Yet, the potential benefits far outweigh the initial apprehension. You're bound to find a sense of comfort and community that can significantly ease the journey through memory issues.

In conclusion, support groups play an instrumental role in the quilt of support systems available to those facing memory problems. They offer emotional sanctuary, practical advice, and a sense of community that is both comforting and empowering. By participating in these groups, you both offer and receive strengths that collectively build a fortification against the challenges posed by memory decline. Taking that first step into a support group could be one of the most affirming actions you can take, providing invaluable assistance on your journey.

CHAPTER 11:
LEGAL AND FINANCIAL
CONSIDERATIONS

As we navigate the terrain of memory issues, addressing legal and financial matters becomes an essential step to ensure peace of mind. It's crucial to plan ahead by setting up necessary legal documents, such as a power of attorney, which appoints a trusted individual to make decisions on your behalf should you be unable to do so. This foresight can safeguard your assets and provide clear directives for your care, easing potential burdens on loved ones. Furthermore, organizing your finances and understanding the benefits you're entitled to, like social security and healthcare options, can significantly reduce stress. Taking these steps early not only secures your future but also provides a comforting assurance, allowing you to focus on enjoying life's moments with clarity and ease.

Planning Ahead

When facing memory issues, it's essential to think about the future and what steps you can take now to make later stages of life simpler and more manageable. The concept of "planning ahead" might feel overwhelming, especially when coupled with the daily challenges that come with memory problems. However, taking time now to put certain elements in place can provide peace of mind and ensure that your wishes are followed concerning your well-being, finances, and legal matters.

First, consider putting together an organized system of important documents. This might include your will, insurance policies, names of family members, and financial records. Keeping these in a safe yet accessible place can significantly reduce the stress and confusion for both you and your loved ones. Labeling folders clearly and making a list of their contents could be incredibly beneficial for those who might be assisting you in the future.

Another crucial step is to designate a durable power of attorney. This is someone you trust to make financial and health-related decisions on your behalf, should the need arise. Choose a person who understands your values and desires, and have a conversation with them about what you expect. This ensures that your intentions are respected even if you're no longer able to communicate them yourself.

Additionally, it's wise to think about setting up an advance healthcare directive. This legal document outlines your preferences for medical treatment and end-of-life care. Discussing your choices with your healthcare provider can clarify options and ensure that your directive includes comprehensive and instructive details. It's vital not only for your peace of mind but also for guiding your loved ones in making emotionally challenging decisions.

Creating a financial strategy tailored to your current and future needs is also part of long-term planning. This might involve budgeting for medical expenses, long-term care, or even day-to-day living costs. Consulting with a financial advisor who understands the complexities associated with aging and memory issues can help secure your financial future.

Having conversations with family members about your financial and legal plans is another key to effective planning. Open dialogue can prevent misunderstandings and ensure everyone knows your wishes. It's essential to clear any potential ambiguities, smoothing the way for those who'll be providing support.

Please remember to continually re-evaluate your plan. Life changes and so do our needs and circumstances. Regularly reviewing your documents and arrangements will keep everything up to date. This reassessment can provide additional reassurance that your plans remain applicable and effective.

Planning ahead isn't just about paperwork and legalities—it's about setting the stage for a more secure and less stressful future. By laying the groundwork now, you're not only protecting your interests but also making things easier for your loved ones who may need to step in down the line. This peace of mind can afford you more energy and clarity to enjoy the present moment, despite the memory issues you may be facing.

Finally, **don't hesitate to seek professional advice** when needed. Many experts are familiar with the unique challenges that come with aging and memory loss, including elder law attorneys, financial planners, and healthcare advisors. They can provide specialized guidance tailored to your situation, helping you navigate the complex landscape of legal and financial planning.

Effective planning is both an act of self-care and a gift to those you trust and cherish. By addressing these considerations early, you're establishing a roadmap that honors your choices and affords you the dignity and respect you deserve. And more importantly, you're taking steps toward a future where memory issues don't define your quality of life. With preparation, compassion, and thoughtful strategy, you can face the years ahead with confidence and tranquility.

Power of Attorney

As we journey through life, it's important to consider the legal and financial aspects that come with aging, especially when facing memory issues. One crucial tool in this planning process is the Power of Attorney (POA). This document ensures that someone you trust can make decisions on your behalf if you're unable to do so. Understanding the intricacies of a Power of Attorney can provide you and your loved ones with peace of mind.

A Power of Attorney is a legal document that grants another person, known as the "agent" or "attorney-in-fact," the authority to act on your behalf. This can encompass a wide range of responsibilities, from managing financial matters to making critical healthcare decisions. This power can be as broad or as specific as you decide, and it can be crucial, especially as memory issues become more pronounced.

There are different types of Power of Attorney, and each serves a unique purpose. A General Power of Attorney grants your agent broad authority to act on your behalf in a variety of matters. Alternatively, a Special or Limited Power of Attorney restricts the agent's power to specific tasks or situations. For individuals facing memory challenges, a Durable Power of Attorney is often the most appropriate. This type remains in effect even if you're incapacitated. Without it, your loved ones might face legal hurdles to step in and help.

Establishing a Power of Attorney early, before significant memory deterioration occurs, is vital. It's easier to discuss and create this document when you're still capable of making sound decisions. Moreover, it avoids putting your family in a position where they must seek guardianship or conservatorship, which can be time-consuming and emotionally taxing.

While choosing your agent, consider someone you trust implicitly. This person should understand your values and be willing to act in your best interest. Typically, people choose close family members or friends as their agents. However, it's essential to have candid conversations with the chosen person to ensure they're comfortable with the responsibility. Detailed guidance and clear communication will aid them in fulfilling your wishes accurately.

Appointing a successor agent can also be a prudent step. If your primary agent is unable or unwilling to serve when the time comes, having a backup ensures that your affairs are continuously managed without interruption. This foresight adds another layer of security to your planning.

Drafting a Power of Attorney isn't something you should do independently. Consulting with an elder law attorney or a knowledgeable legal expert is highly recommended. They can tailor the document to fit your specific needs, adhering to state laws and avoiding potential legal pitfalls. This professional guidance is invaluable in creating a document that stands up to scrutiny and serves your best interests.

Healthcare decisions are another critical area where a Power of Attorney can play a role. A Healthcare Power of Attorney, also known as a Medical Power of Attorney, allows your agent to make medical decisions if you're unable. This is particularly important for those experiencing significant memory loss. It ensures that someone who knows your health care preferences can advocate for you, maintaining your autonomy even when your memory might fail you.

In addition to a Power of Attorney, including an Advance Healthcare Directive or Living Will can provide further clarity. These documents specify your wishes regarding life-sustaining treatment and other healthcare preferences. When used in conjunction, they give a comprehensive view of your desires, guiding your healthcare agent effectively.

It's equally important to revisit and potentially update your Power of Attorney as circumstances change. Regular reviews can ensure that the document reflects your current wishes and that the appointed agent is still the best choice for your evolving situation. If your relationship with your agent changes, or if they become unable to serve, updating the Power of Attorney will ensure that your affairs remain in capable hands.

Communication with relevant parties is essential once your Power of Attorney is in place. Inform your doctors, financial institutions, and other significant entities of your agent's role. Providing them with copies of the document can facilitate smoother transitions when your agent needs to act on your behalf. Transparency in these matters can prevent complications and ensure your agent's directives are honored promptly.

Furthermore, it's beneficial to keep the original Power of Attorney document in a secure but accessible place. Informing your agent and close family members of its location can prevent delays in accessing the document when needed. Keeping an additional copy with your elder law attorney or a trusted individual adds an extra layer of security.

For many, setting up a Power of Attorney can seem daunting, but breaking down the process into manageable steps helps. Starting with thorough discussions with your loved ones, followed by seeking legal advice, and finally formalizing the document, can make the process straightforward and less intimidating.

In conclusion, a Power of Attorney is a powerful tool in your legal and financial planning arsenal, especially when facing memory issues. It ensures your preferences are honored, provides a roadmap for your loved ones, and safeguards your autonomy. Taking the time to establish and communicate this document is an act of foresight and care for both yourself and those who may need to step in to support you.

CHAPTER 12:
LOOKING FORWARD

As we look forward, it's important to embrace the changes that come with aging and memory issues. Life doesn't stop with a diagnosis; rather, it presents a new way to experience and navigate the world. Finding joy in small moments, staying engaged with family and friends, and remaining positive can reshape your perspective on what lies ahead. Remember, there are countless strategies and support systems out there to help you maintain a fulfilling and meaningful life. Don't worry about doing everything perfectly; celebrate your successes, big and small. Aging and memory issues require adjustment, but with the right mindset and resources, you can look forward to each day with hope and resilience.

Embracing Change

Change is an inevitable part of life, and when it comes to facing memory issues, such a reality can feel particularly daunting. However, embracing change does not mean surrendering to it; rather, it involves adapting and finding resilience within oneself. Change can be an opportunity for growth and self-discovery, even when it is unexpected or challenging.

It's essential to understand that the process of adapting to memory issues is not a linear journey. There will be days of frustration and confusion, interspersed with moments of clarity and success. Embracing change means accepting these fluctuations and finding the strength to move forward despite them. This adaptive outlook enables not only the individual but also their families and caregivers to navigate the complexities of memory-related conditions with greater ease and understanding.

One key aspect of embracing change involves a willingness to be open to new strategies and solutions. Technology, for instance, offers a plethora of tools designed to assist those coping with memory issues. From simple reminder apps to more sophisticated cognitive training platforms, there is a wide range of options to help maintain independence and improve quality of life. Do not shy away from exploring these tools, as they can significantly aid in making daily activities more manageable.

Equally important is the role of social support. Surrounding oneself with a network of compassionate and understanding individuals can make a substantial difference. Whether it's family, friends, or support groups, these connections provide emotional reassurance and practical assistance. Engaging in open dialogues about your experience can dismantle feelings of isolation, making the journey less burdensome.

Maintaining an active and healthy lifestyle also facilitates positive adaptation to memory changes. Regular physical activity, a balanced diet, and good sleep hygiene collectively contribute to improved cognitive function and overall well-being. Incorporating these habits may require adjustments, but the benefits extend far beyond the physical realm, enhancing emotional stability and fostering a sense of empowerment.

Moreover, cultivating a mindset that is both accepting and forward-looking is invaluable. Life with memory issues will indeed have its set of challenges, but it's also filled with opportunities to discover strengths and capabilities that may have previously been overlooked. Reflecting on past achievements can be a source of motivation, reminding you that resilience has always been part of your character.

It's also beneficial to recognize that memory issues typically progress gradually. This gradual evolution means there is time to adapt, learn, and implement new strategies. Making small, incremental changes rather than attempting drastic overhauls can lead to more sustainable adjustments. Incremental changes also provide the space to celebrate small victories, which are crucial for maintaining morale and a positive outlook.

There's a profound power in viewing each day as a chance to embrace the new normal. This mindset shift encourages one to find joy in small, everyday moments and reinforces the value of staying engaged with life's tapestry. Activities that might have seemed mundane before—such as gardening, reading, or spending time with loved ones—can take on new meaning and importance. Taking pleasure in these activities can greatly enhance quality of life and provide a sense of accomplishment.

It's worth mentioning that creativity can be a significant ally in this journey. Engaging in creative endeavors like painting, knitting, or writing can serve as both a therapeutic outlet and a way to exercise the brain. These activities can become a form of self-expression that conveys feelings and experiences words might not be able to encapsulate fully. Furthermore, creativity often brings joy and satisfaction, elements essential for combating the emotional impact of memory issues.

In the broader societal context, there is a growing awareness and acceptance of memory issues, which helps reduce stigma and fosters a more inclusive environment. Advances in medical research and public health initiatives are continuously being made, providing hope for more effective treatments and support mechanisms. Being informed about these advancements can imbue a sense of optimism and active engagement with one's own well-being.

It's also helpful to explore mindfulness and meditation. These practices help in grounding the mind and alleviating stress, which can be particularly beneficial when dealing with the uncertainties brought by memory changes. Techniques such as focused breathing and mindful observation of one's thoughts can bring clarity and calmness, facilitating a better emotional response to daily challenges.

Lastly, embracing change necessitates a degree of patience—with oneself and with the process. There will be moments of exasperation and self-doubt, but these should be met with compassion and understanding. Allowing oneself the grace to experience these emotions without judgment fosters a healthier mental state and enhances the ability to adapt.

In summation, embracing change in the context of memory issues involves a mixture of openness, adaptability, and resilience. It asks for an acceptance of the new reality, a willingness to explore new tools and strategies, and the cultivation of a supportive network. Through this multifaceted approach, it's possible to lead a fulfilling and meaningful life, even in the face of memory challenges. Embracing this journey not only transforms the experience but also paves the way for discovering newfound strengths and joys.

Staying Positive

Maintaining a positive outlook when facing memory issues can feel like a daunting task. However, it is possible and could even improve your overall quality of life. Embracing a positive mindset doesn't mean ignoring the challenges that come with memory problems. Instead, it involves finding ways to adapt and flourish despite the difficulties. A positive attitude can go a long way in helping you manage your memory issues.

The first step in staying positive involves acknowledging your current capabilities and accepting where you are. It's easy to get caught up in what you've lost or what may become harder to do. But instead of dwelling on these aspects, focus on what you can still do and the strengths you possess. Celebrating small victories and being grateful for what remains functional in your life can set the stage for a more positive outlook.

One practical approach to fostering positivity is through maintaining social connections. Interacting with loved ones and participating in social activities can lift your spirits and keep you connected. Whether it's joining a book club, having regular coffee dates with friends, or attending community events, remaining socially engaged can bring joy and a sense of belonging. No one should face memory issues alone; lean on your community and family for support.

Engaging in activities that bring you joy and stimulate your mind can also be a tremendous boost. Whether it's gardening, painting, or playing a musical instrument, these hobbies can serve as a therapeutic escape and provide a sense of accomplishment. Activities that require focus, creativity, and problem-solving can even help in maintaining cognitive functions. The key is to find what you love and dive into it with enthusiasm.

Nurturing a sense of purpose can be very empowering. Many find comfort in volunteering, mentoring, or even sharing their own journey with others who are facing similar challenges. Feeling like you're making a difference and contributing to the well-being of others can significantly enhance your outlook on life. Purpose can be a potent antidote to feelings of helplessness or frustration that sometimes accompany memory issues.

Laughter and humor are often overlooked aspects of positivity. It's true what they say: laughter is the best medicine. Watching a funny movie, reading a humorous book, or simply sharing a laugh with friends can lighten your mood and alleviate stress. Humor can serve as a gentle reminder that, despite our problems, there's still joy to be found in everyday moments.

In addition, don't underestimate the importance of physical health in maintaining a positive mindset. Regular exercise, a balanced diet, and adequate sleep not only benefit physical health but also mental well-being. Physical activity releases endorphins, which are natural mood lifters. Good nutrition fuels both body and mind, while adequate sleep helps in regulating mood and cognitive functions. Taking care of your body can, in turn, help you stay mentally positive.

Another tool in your positivity toolkit can be mindfulness and meditation. These practices can help ground you in the present moment, reducing anxieties about the future and regrets about the past. Simple breathing exercises, guided meditations, or even quiet moments of reflection can create a state of calmness and clarity. This mental clarity can assist you in handling daily challenges more effectively.

Engaging with inspirational content can provide a wellspring of positivity. Reading books that uplift your spirit, watching motivational talks, or listening to music that moves you can ignite a sense of hope and encouragement. Sometimes, external inspiration can rekindle internal motivation, guiding you through tougher days.

It's crucial to also allow yourself space to feel and process emotions. There will be days when staying positive feels like an uphill battle, and it's alright to acknowledge these feelings. Emotional honesty is integral to mental wellness; trying to suppress feelings can often lead to more stress. Share your feelings with trusted friends, family, or a professional counselor. Expressing your thoughts can be incredibly liberating and can pave the way back to a more positive frame of mind.

Setting realistic goals and celebrating incremental progress helps in maintaining a positive outlook. Instead of overwhelming yourself with unrealistic expectations, break your tasks into smaller, achievable steps. Each small victory can build momentum and provide a sense of accomplishment. Over time, these tiny steps can lead to significant improvements in both mood and daily functioning.

Lastly, remember the power of gratitude. Engaging in a daily practice of reflecting on things you're thankful for can dramatically shift your perspective. Creating a gratitude journal where you jot down three positive things about each day is a simple yet powerful exercise. It helps to light up your focus on life's positives, diminishing the weight of its challenges.

Overall, staying positive while dealing with memory issues involves a multi-faceted approach encompassing emotional acceptance, social engagement, physical health, mindfulness, and purposeful activity. It's a journey that requires patience, flexibility, and self-compassion. By embracing these strategies, you're not only managing your memory issues but also enriching your life in meaningful ways.

Above all, remember that it's okay to ask for help. Support is always around the corner, be it from family, friends, or professional services. Embracing assistance doesn't signify weakness; rather, it highlights your strength and determination to navigate through life's complexities while cherishing its joys.

As you continue this journey, let the essence of positivity guide you, enrich your days, and bring light to the moments that truly matter. Your journey is unique, and so are your strengths. Cherish them, lean on them, and let them propel you forward. The future may hold uncertainties, but with a positive mindset, you are equipped to face them with grace and resilience.

CONCLUSION

As we reach the conclusion of this journey, it's crucial to remember that experiencing memory issues does not signify an end but rather a transformation. Memory changes are a natural part of aging and do not have to diminish your quality of life. Instead, they can serve as an invitation to explore new ways of engaging with the world around you.

Memory challenges can seem daunting, leading to feelings of frustration or sadness. However, armed with knowledge and the right support, you can navigate these changes effectively. Consider the techniques and strategies discussed throughout this book—each one is a tool designed to empower you. From understanding the intricacies of the aging brain and recognizing early signs, to exploring various treatment options and making important lifestyle adjustments, each chapter aimed to equip you with valuable insights.

It is vital to maintain open communication with your loved ones and healthcare providers. Honest conversations can ease the burden and foster a sense of community. No one should face these challenges alone, and by reaching out, you create a network of support that can provide both practical assistance and emotional comfort.

Implementing simple strategies into your daily routine can make a significant difference. Establishing consistent routines, using technological aids, and incorporating engaging activities can enhance your day-to-day life. These small changes can accumulate into noticeable improvements in your memory and overall well-being.

Consider the importance of a balanced lifestyle. Diet, exercise, sleep, and stress management play pivotal roles in maintaining cognitive health. By prioritizing these aspects, you not only support your memory functions but also improve your overall health, enabling you to live more fully and joyfully.

Legal and financial planning provides peace of mind, allowing you to focus on living positively rather than worrying about the future. Establishing documents like power of attorney and advance directives ensure your wishes are respected, and your needs are met, freeing you to concentrate on the aspects of life that bring you happiness and fulfillment.

Above all, facing memory issues with a positive attitude can transform your experience. Embracing change and continually finding new ways to connect with your environment can lead to profound personal growth. It is a journey of adaptation, discovery, and resilience.

Remember that memory loss doesn't define your worth or your contribution to your family and society. Your wisdom, experiences, and presence remain invaluable. You are not alone in this experience; many resources and communities are dedicated to supporting you every step of the way.

In closing, let this book be a reminder of the strength within you and the vast array of options available to help manage memory issues effectively. It's a call to action to embrace your journey with hope and determination and to recognize that life, with all its challenges, continues to offer beauty and joy.

Take each day as it comes, cherish the moments, and lean on the supportive structures around you. Your journey with memory issues is not an end but a new chapter of life filled with potential and growth.

APPENDIX A:
APPENDIX

W e've walked through many aspects of understanding memory issues, from the early signs to treatment options and daily living tips, always with the goal of providing clarity and support. This appendix aims to offer additional resources and important contacts to help you or your loved ones continue on this journey with confidence and reassurance.

Resources for Further Reading

- **Books**
    - *"The Aging Brain: Proven Steps to Prevent Dementia and Sharpen Your Mind"* by Dr. Timothy R. Jennings
    - *"Still Alice"* by Lisa Genova
    - *"The End of Alzheimer's: The First Program to Prevent and Reverse Cognitive Decline"* by Dr. Dale Bredesen
    - *"Creating Moments of Joy Along the Alzheimer's Journey"* by Jolene Brackey

- **Websites**
    - Alzheimer's Association - Information and resources on Alzheimer's and dementia.
    - National Institute on Aging - Comprehensive research and resources on aging and memory.
    - BrightFocus Foundation - Updates on research and strategies for Alzheimer's disease.

- UCSF Memory and Aging Center - Resources for patients and caregivers dealing with neurodegenerative diseases.

Contact Information for Support Organizations

- **Alzheimer's Association**

Phone: 1-800-272-3900

Website: https://www.alz.org

- **National Institute on Aging**

Phone: 1-800-222-2225

Website: https://www.nia.nih.gov

- **BrightFocus Foundation**

Phone: 1-800-437-2423

Website: https://www.brightfocus.org

- **UCSF Memory and Aging Center**

Phone: 1-415-353-2057

Website: https://www.memoryandagingcenter.org

As you continue to navigate the complexities of memory issues, don't hesitate to reach out to these organizations. They provide valuable information, support networks, and tools that can make a significant difference in daily life.

Remember, understanding and addressing memory issues is a journey. It's a path walked with empathy, knowledge, and above all, hope. The resources and contacts provided here are your companions on this journey, guiding and supporting you every step of the way.

www.ingramcontent.com/pod-product-compliance
Lightning Source LLC
Chambersburg PA
CBHW031124180526
45160CB00001B/14